CROSSING
THE
HEALING ZONE

From Illness to Wellness

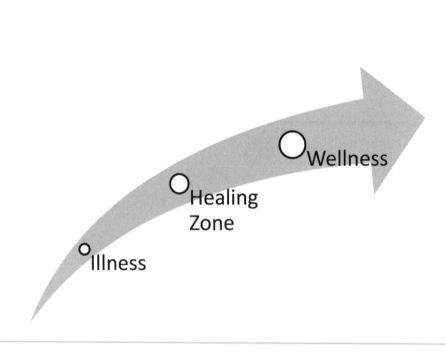

CROSSING
THE
HEALING
ZONE

From Illness to Wellness

Ashok Bedi, M.D.

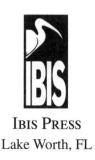

IBIS PRESS
Lake Worth, FL

Published in 2013 by Ibis Press
A division of Nicolas-Hays, Inc.
P. O. Box 540206
Lake Worth, FL 33454-0206
www.ibispress.net

Distributed to the trade by
Red Wheel/Weiser, LLC
65 Parker St. • Ste. 7
Newburyport, MA 01950
www.redwheelweiser.com

ISBN 978-0-89254-203-1

Library of Congress Cataloging-in-Publication Data
Bedi, Ashok.
 Crossing the healing zone : from illness to wellness / Ashok Bedi, M.D.
      pages cm
   Summary: "Crossing the Healing Zone: From Illness to Wellness advances the
new concepts of the emerging frontiers of integrative medicine, merging East
and West, Body, Mind and Soul with a Jungian perspective guided by Arche-
types and Myths, Active Imagination, Dreams and Synchronicities in explor-
ing the neuroplastic mysteries of the Healing Zone. His book is focused on the
Mind, Body, Soul and Spirit connection"-- Provided by publisher.
   Includes bibliographical references and index.
   ISBN 978-0-89254-203-1 (pbk.)
   1. Alternative medicine. 2. Integrative medicine. 3. Mind and body. I. Title.
   R733.B436 2013
   616--dc23   2012048762

Book design and production by Studio 31
www.studio31.com

Printed in the United States of America
(MG)

Contents

Acknowledgments

This book was inspired by the wisdom of the ancient rishis—the holy men and women of India—as well as by contemporary rishis of our own culture, including His Holiness the Dalai Lama, Guruji Shree B. K. S. Iyengar, Carl G. Jung, Deepak Chopra, Richard Davidson, Shree Bhante Henepola Gurnaratana, Herbert Benson, and Jon Kabat-Zinn.

Many thanks to the following authors and publishers for permission to quote from their books and sources: Micha Lindemans for permission to reprint material from *Encyclopedia Mythica* (*pantheon.org*); the International Gita Society for their kind permission to use quotes from *Bhagwad Gita;* Charles Haynes and Hoysala temple for the Narshima image that was adapted for this book (*http://creativecommons.org*).

I am grateful to the graphic artists Harshad Kamdar (*www.photografix.us*), Karen Higgins, and the late John Peters for many of the graphics in this book; to photographer Alyssa Otter (*www.dgxstudio.com*) for the author photograph; and to my daughter, Ami Bedi, for her support and guidance during several trips to India to the Goddess sites to collect stories, photographs, and inspiration. The yantra images in the book are adapted from the excellent images created by Per Krueger at the Swedish Institute of Computer Science (see *http://www.sics.se/~piak/yoga/yantra/*).

Several of my colleagues have contributed to the making of this book. The Appendix (Physics and the Psyche) was written in collaboration with my brother, Dr. Alkesh Punjabi, Professor of Physics and Mathematics at Hampton University. Much of the material on brain-wave training was contributed by my trusted colleague, neurofeedback expert and clinical psychologist Dr. David Drapes. My colleague Bonnie Cleveland helped define my thinking on the contribution of Level 5 response to our fight-or-flight instinct (Cannon, 1915). My grandson, Signe, and my colleague and friend Dr.

Dinshah Gagrat kindly compiled their favorite music playlists upon my request to contribute to this book.

I am also grateful to my grandson for helping me develop many of my ideas during our frequent evening walks together. He often challenged me with an outside-the-box view of my ideas and motivated me to explore them from a totally unique perspective. I am grateful to my editor, David Luhrssen, for taking a dry academic treatise and transforming it into a book that is accessible to a broad audience and to seekers of the soul. My copy editor Laurel Warren Trufant, Ph.D. at ProLogos Editorial Services made the manuscript eminently more concise and focused. Finally, my special thanks to my patients who challenged my ideas in my clinical field test of these concepts and helped me refine them to the point of relevance in their recovery and healing.

I have also drawn from the thinking and research of many writers and physicians through their published works. Many of these are listed in the bibliography at the end of this book. If I have inadvertently missed someone, I apologize in advance and will be honored to rectify the error in reprints of the book. My special thanks to the Jungian analysts Murray Stein in Zurich, David H. Rosen in Texas, Donald Kalsched in New York, Marvin J. Spiegelman in Los Angles, Boris Matthews in Madison, and the late Arwind U. Vasavada from Chicago for inspiring me over the years with their unique contributions to contemporary Jungian thought.

Introduction

In the 20th century, medicine was strictly concerned with treating illnesses. The medicine of the 21st century is about wellness. Medical science continues to make strides, harvesting the dividends of emerging technology in the service of detection and treatment. However, we have reached a tipping point where the emphasis is shifting toward the wellness that emerges from living life to our highest potential. Inseparable from this trend is a renewed respect for and interest in ancient healing systems, which are being reinterpreted and reconfigured to create the integrative medicine of the future. With the help of new technology, we are now able to subject our ancestral wisdom to the rigors of evidence-based medicine and assimilate the best of these traditions into a healthy way of life.

What I call the Healing Zone, which lies between illness and wellness, is fraught with dangers and is treacherous to navigate. We can easily be swept away in the vortex where psychology and spirituality converge with our physical bodies. You can cross the Healing Zone under the guidance of qualified professionals like acupuncturists, Ayurvedic physicians, Chinese medicine specialists, chiropractors, homeopaths, naturopaths, herbalists, hypnotherapists, and massage therapists. However, there are other safe fording places that you can identify and use to cross the Healing Zone in your own daily life and practice. The goal of this book is to inform and empower you—to make you aware of these crossing points in the flow of the Healing Zone so that you can become an active partner in the process of moving from illness to wellness. We will also discuss the theory and practice of using these crossing points.

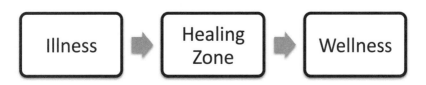

Contemporary Western medicine is disease-based and focuses on the work of specialists rather than generalists. It is reactive rather than proactive, crisis-oriented rather than holistic, physician-directed rather than interactive, and focused on curing illnesses rather than promoting wellness. Medical treatment is delivered via a chaotic, disconnected matrix of urgent-care facilities, emergency rooms, hospitals, and specialists. The presumed driver of this care, the family physician, is at the bottom of this pyramid.

The emerging integrative medicine of the 21st century will be patient-focused, empowering individuals to take care of themselves through a balanced lifestyle that uses their unique personal resources and attributes, and invokes the traditions of their ancestral wisdom and their souls' guidance. In this model, patients will map out, not only their illness profiles, but also their wellness plans. In this new paradigm, the emphasis is on accessing the Healing Zone to move from a focus on illness to a goal of enhancing wellness.

According to the National Center for Complementary Medicine, 42 percent of Americans use at least some of the methods of wellness medicine we will discuss (Spiegel, 2003). More patients visit practitioners of these complementary methods of treatment than visit primary-care doctors. Among the main reasons for seeking these alternatives are pain, pediatrics, and self-care for stress and weight loss. Fifty percent of cancer patients and AIDS survivors consult complementary-care providers. Seventy-two percent of these patients don't talk about it with their doctors, yet studies show that 83 percent of patients combine alternative with conventional medicine.

The Healing Zone is a place of awe and mystery. It is not a linear phenomenon, but a quantum field where energy and matter become interchangeable. This book will explore the neuroplastic mysteries of the Healing Zone and lay the foundation for discussing the stress and rejuvenation systems of your body, the archetypes and myths that guide you across the flow of the Healing Zone, and specific practices that are accessible to most of us. These include cultivating a spiritual attitude, "Googling" the unconscious with your dreams and synchronicities, using active-imagination techniques, working with your complexes, hang-ups, fascinations, and antipathies, reconfiguring your cognitive distortions to deal with addictive cravings, and linking mandala therapy with neurofeedback. We will also explore more traditional disciplines like pranayama, yoga, meditation, mindfulness attitude and practice, music, yantra techniques, and Kundalini balancing. With some instruction, these methods may help you to navigate the Healing Zone from illness to wellness.

Some of these methods are so much a part of the fabric of our self-healing system that we use them intuitively, without being aware of it. The most common form of self-healing is prayer, while the least common is humor; there is emerging evidence that both are therapeutic. Some writers propose that we may be "wired for God" (Foster, 2011), while others speculate that we may have a "God gene" (Hamer, 2005). According to *Scientific American* reviewer Carl Zimmer, Hamer looked at the DNA samples of some of his subjects, hoping to find variants of genes that tended to turn up in self-transcendent people. His search led him to a gene known as VMAT2. Two different versions of this gene exist, differing only at a single position. People with one version of the gene tend to score a little higher on self-transcendence tests. Although the influence is small, it is, Hamer claims, consistent. About half the people in the study had at least one copy of the self-transcendence-boosting version of VMAT2, "the God gene." Others (Alper, 2008) propose that humanity's perception of a spiritual realm is actually the biological result of thousands of years of evolution. In other words, the God gene is "nature's white lie"—a coping mechanism selected into our species to help alleviate the debilitating anxiety caused by our unique awareness of death.

Two academics at the University of Pennsylvania's Center for Spirituality and the Mind contend that contemplating God actually reduces stress, which in turn prevents the deterioration of the brain's dendrites and increases neuroplasticity. The authors conclude that meditation and other spiritual practices permanently strengthen neural functioning in specific parts of the brain that aid in lowering anxiety and depression, thus enhancing social awareness and empathy and improving cognitive functioning (Waldman, 2009).

Of course, the role of religion, spirituality, community, and prayer in health has been a subject of debate for a long time. The Roseto study (Bruhn, 1998) investigated the striking differences in mortality from myocardial infarction between Roseto, a homogeneous Italian-American community in Pennsylvania, and other nearby towns between 1955 and 1965. These differences disappeared as Roseto became more "Americanized" in the 1960s. A more recent study (Egolf, 1992) extended the comparison over a longer period of time to test the hypothesis that the findings from this period were not due to random fluctuations in small communities. The researchers examined death certificates for Roseto and Bangor from 1935 to 1985. Age-standardized death rates and mortality ratios were computed for each decade. They found that the Rosetans had a lower mortality rate from myocardial infarction over the course of the first thirty years, but that mortality rose to the level of Bangor's following a period of erosion of traditional cohesive family and community relationships. This mortality-rate increase involved mainly younger Rosetan men and elderly women. The data confirmed the existence of consistent mortality differences between Roseto and Bangor during a time when there were many indicators of greater social solidarity and homogeneity in Roseto.

The unanswered question in the Roseto study was whether the differences in mortality rates in the two towns were related to community or religion. A further study (Kark, 1996) emphasized that religious observance had a strong positive influence on protecting health. This study assessed the association of Jewish religious observance with mortality by comparing religious and secular kibbutzim. These collectives are highly similar in social structure and economic function and are cohesive and supportive communities. A sixteen-year (1970–1985) study of mortality in eleven religious and eleven secular kibbutzim found that mortality was considerably higher in secular kibbutzim. The lower mortality in religious kibbutzim was consistent for all major causes of death.

Another study (Randolph, 1988) found a positive therapeutic effect from intercessory prayer in coronary-care patients. The therapeutic effects of prayer, one of the oldest forms of therapy, have had little attention in the medical literature. To evaluate the effects in a coronary-care unit (CCU) population, a prospective randomized double-blind protocol was followed. Over ten months, 393 patients admitted to the CCU were randomized, after signing informed consent, to an intercessory prayer group or to a control group. While hospitalized, the first group received intercessory prayer by participating Christians praying outside the hospital; the control group did not. At entry, analysis revealed no statistical difference between the groups. After entry, all patients were followed for the remainder of the admission. The prayer group subsequently had significantly better results, while patients in the control group required ventilatory assistance, antibiotics, and diuretics more frequently. According to Randolph, this data suggests that intercessory prayer to the Judeo-Christian God has a beneficial therapeutic effect in patients admitted to a CCU.

The gist of this debate was well summarized by Carl Jung in his communication to Bill W., the founder of Alcoholics Anonymous, who acknowledged Jung's contribution to AA's methods. Bill W. wanted to acknowledge AA's debt to those who contributed to its creation (W., 1988). In his letter of January 23, 1961, he traced the story of Rowland H., who, having exhausted all treatment efforts for his alcoholism, became Jung's patient for a year (1931) and showed much improvement. However, he soon relapsed and returned to Jung as a last resort. Jung confronted him with the hopelessness of his situation and the futility of any further treatment options, with the possible exception of some religious or spiritual experience.

Shortly thereafter, Rowland joined the Oxford Group, an evangelical movement in Europe that emphasized the principles of self-survey, confession, restitution, and service to others. After his conversion experience released him from his alcoholism, Rowland returned to New York and helped Edwin T. (Ebby) to achieve sobriety. Ebby inspired Bill W. to seek his own recovery by acknowledging the collapse of his ego followed by a spiritual experience. Ebby gave Bill W. a copy of William James' *Varieties of Religious Experience* (James, 1988), which explores this conversion process. With the guidance of his physician, Dr. William Silkworth, Bill W. went on to establish Alcoholics Anonymous.

In his response to Bill W. on January 30, 1961 (W., 1988), Jung identified an alcoholic or addict's craving as a low-level equivalent of our spiritual thirst for wholeness—a union with God. In Latin, alcohol is called *spiritus*. Thus the same word is used for the highest religious experience and a potentially depraving poison. The helpful formula therefore is: *spiritus contra spiritum*.

In my own analytical and clinical experience, I have found that our medical and psychiatric problems—our complexes and hang-ups, our accidents and synchronicities, our relationship tangles with friends and foe alike, our dreams and creative processes— are manifestations of a yearning for connection with this *spiritus* (Bedi, 2000). The path from illness to wellness is a search for Spirit via the Healing Zone.

Humor is the most neglected crossing point in the Healing Zone. Humor is the tendency of particular cognitive experiences to provoke laughter and provide amusement. The term derives from the *humoral* medicine of the ancient Greeks, which taught that the balance of fluids known as humors in the human body (Latin: *húmor*, "body fluid") controls human health and emotion. Norman Cousins (Cousins, 1979), editor of *The Saturday Review*, cured himself of an unknown illness with a self-invented regimen of laughter and vitamins. Many recent studies have examined the therapeutic benefits of humor (Berk, 1989; Joshua, 2005; Penson, 2005; Seaward, 1992; Weisenberg, 1995; Ziegler, 1995).

Each section of this book will discuss the psychology and the science behind one suggested method of crossing the Healing Zone, followed by practical words of wisdom and exercises that can be part of your personal wellness program.

Chapter 1

The Mystery and Science
of the Healing Zone

Our minds and bodies are always in flux. Stress poses a constant threat by triggering a negative flow, while our systems continuously attempt to create a positive flow to enhance health and well-being. In recent years, stress has been identified as a significant health problem. A healthy response to stress leads to vitality, joy, and peace. An unhealthy response results in disease, dysfunction, and a diminished participation in love, work, play, creativity, and spirituality.

There are fundamental differences between East and West in dealing with stress. While the West has made significant strides in material progress and mastery of the immediate environment, the East offers much wisdom for achieving health, happiness, and wholeness, including the skillful management of stress. When East and West collaborate, all of humanity will benefit from an integrated approach to healing illness and enjoying the gifts of a soulful life. This book offers a path toward that integration, with the objective of helping you heal the suffering of your mind, your body, your soul, and your relationships. Eastern spiritual wisdom and the Western intellectual tradition are the yin and the yang of your consciousness. When they do their dance together, they create the Healing Zone.

The Fourth Dimension of Consciousness

The Indian healing system recognizes four states of experience—wakefulness, dreaming, dreamless deep sleep, and a transitional state that connects the others. The first three are distinct, as evidenced by brain recordings during these states. More advanced brain-imaging techniques have confirmed what rishis and wise men and women in the East have known for thousands of years—that there is a fourth state connecting the other three. The process of transition between these states has always intrigued Easterners. What happens to our minds, brains, bodies, and souls when we are in transit?

The transitional space in which this occurs is the fourth dimension of our existence, where we are neither awake or asleep or dreaming, but suspended in the void, the realm of the goddess Aditi, whom we will discuss later (see figure 1). When we engage this void, we can create new consciousness with the help of the healing wisdom of the universe. The meditative and contemplative practices of all the great traditions—including Buddhist mindfulness, transcendental meditation, Christian contemplative practices, and yoga—help us engage this void and its healing potential. When suspended in this void, we are in direct communion with the healing energy of Spirit and the wisdom of the universe.

However, most of these practices are one-way streets—methods in which we passively receive healing wisdom. The great psychoanalyst Carl Jung made a giant leap forward in dealing with the fourth dimension of consciousness when he invented a method for engaging this void actively. He coined the term "active imagination" to describe this method.

According to the Hindu scriptures, when a young soul becomes an old soul worthy of merging with Spirit (the collective consciousness), it is in a state called *moksha*. Moksha means freedom from the cycles of life and death, liberation from reincarnation, and transcendence of the opposite tendencies in our nature, personalities, and psyches. In moksha, the Atman (the individual soul) merges with the Brahmana (the collective consciousness or Spirit) much as a drop of water merges with the ocean. However, when we consciously connect with the healing energy and wisdom of the universe in the Healing Zone, the ocean is absorbed into the drop. This

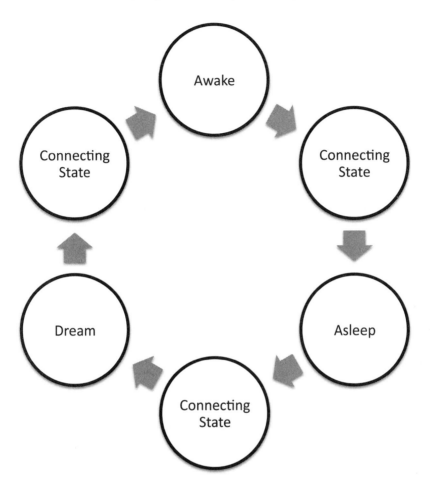

Figure 1. The fourth dimension of consciousness.

is the experience of *ananda*, bliss, *samadhi,* and other manifestations of the fourth state of consciousness.

Psychotherapy becomes another example of crossing the Healing Zone when a therapist raises an aspect of the unconscious into consciousness and maintains this juxtaposition long enough for the experience to be assimilated into consciousness. The insight arrived at during psychotherapy can light the way to a new consciousness and a fundamental transformation of our bodies, minds, psyches, and souls, and the spiritual purpose of our lives. Research by Nobel laureate Eric Kandel (Kandel, 2009) has determined that new learning can change the synapses in a creature as small as a snail.

Quantum Consciousness

When we are in the fourth state of consciousness, we are in a quantum state where mind and body, matter and energy, are readily interchangeable in a fluid continuum. Tremendous transformation is possible in this state of possibility and danger. Here, thoughts, feelings, intuitions, mental images, or memories can be transformed into physical symptoms. Moreover, for therapeutic and healing purposes, the process can be reversed. Psychosomatic symptoms or illnesses can be traced to their primal thoughts, ideas, feelings, or intuitions and made accessible to consciousness. With that insight begins a transformation that results in changes in attitude, feeling, thought, and behavior that eliminate the symptom or illness. This opens the way to a union between ego and soul, and a joining of soul with Spirit.

During the 20th century, Western science dropped many of its objections to ancient Indian beliefs in the nature of consciousness. It dispelled the false notions it had entertained about the nature of matter, which it had defined as that which has mass, weight, and inertia. Science in the age of Einstein and Heisenberg has conceded that the elements of matter are in a state of spontaneous and perpetual motion. In fact, we now know that the most general phenomenon of the universe is vibration, to which the human body and everything else is subject. Various vibrations affect each organ of sensation. Vibrations of a certain quality and number denote to the skin the degree of external temperature; others incite the eye to see different colors; yet others enable the ear to hear defined sounds.

These vibrations can be transmitted by our nervous system with the help of chemical messengers called neurotransmitters.

Science now admits that its previous concept of matter is insufficient to explain many phenomena—for instance, light. Many scientists now believe that there is a substance called ether—a medium that fills the universe and transports, by its vibrations, the radiations of light, heat, electricity, and perhaps action from a distance. The attraction exercised between heavenly bodies may be an example of this.

On further review of the fourth dimension, more details emerge. An individual who is in the Healing Zone and holds two or more levels of consciousness for long enough becomes an alchemical vessel that alters the content of these different modes of consciousness. The emerging mental state may be experienced as an image, an intuition, an insight, or a creative product that has a transformative impact on the individual. This transformation may be positive or negative, numinous or demonic, depending on the integrity and intent of the seeker, his or her level of psychological preparedness, and the skill, perseverance, and guidance available to the aspirant seeking the treasures of the psyche. When divers delve into the ocean depths, they may harvest hidden treasures, or they may be engulfed by the creatures of the deep.

The longer we hold more than two dimensions of consciousness in this alchemic vessel, the more the Healing Zone is activated. The resulting energy matrix leads to a greater quantum soup of mind, matter, energy, soul, Spirit, and cosmic energy. Exponential healing and transformation become possible. In mindfulness, we zoom in on a small object or corner of reality while blocking other aspects of consciousness or reality. In yoga postures, we focus on the body and its connection with the soul and Sprit and exclude all distractions. *Pranayama*, the yoga of breath regulation, involves concentrating on breathing to limit distractions from other aspects of consciousness. In meditation, we focus on a single thought or object to limit conscious or unconscious distraction. Symptoms and problems are dissolved to their origins in the Healing Zone and changed from problems to potential, guiding individuals with a spiritual purposefulness and moving them from ego servitude to the soul path.

In my clinical experience, I have used various methods to make the Healing Zone more accessible. One approach I use is to tune into the consciousness of patients during a session, focusing on their breathing rhythms and synchronizing my own breath with theirs. By doing this, I can influence their physical pain and help them move from pain to bliss or joy. By tuning into a patient's breathing irregularities caused by stress, I can experience both the breathing disturbance and the stress that caused it. Then, by steadying my own breath, my regulated and relaxed breath pattern can be transmitted to the patient, who then experiences more relaxed breathing, which relieves the stress. This is called the *pranic* healing method.

There are other ways to activate the Healing Zone as well— for instance, by tuning into someone's emotional state or physical symptoms. This may be the mechanism for empathy, which has a considerable healing effect. Since the dawn of time, mothers have used this method to tune into their children's mental and physical states. Shamans use similar methods and modern-day psychotherapy intuitively uses this approach without realizing it.

The Psychoid Space

Jung was fascinated by the properties of the Healing Zone, which he called the "pyschoid space" (Jung, 1960). This concept was a precursor of the triune model of the brain discussed later in this book. Jung explained the psychoid space as the gap or flow between our brains and our spiritual dimension (see figure 2). As humans, we are suspended in this gap—the transitional dimension of consciousness between body and Spirit. Our bodies pro-

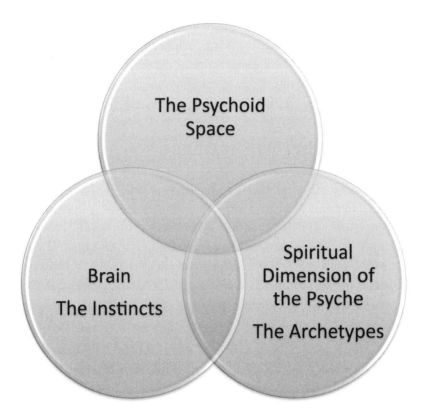

Figure 2. The psychoid space.

vide us with our instincts, while Spirit provides the purpose for our enterprises. For example, nature gives a woman beautiful breasts; Spirit guides her to engage her breasts in erotic life and maternal nurturance, under the guidance of the archetypes Eros and Magna Mater, the Great Mother. Jung describes this duality in consciousness as the red zone and the blue zone. The red zone encompasses the reptilian, instinctual, embodied aspects of our inner lives; the blue zone embraces the spiritual purpose of the psyche. The red zone is the boiler room of the psyche, generating energy; the blue zone is the navigation system that guides the psyche to its eventual purpose. Under the influence of the red zone, the breasts engage the lover and a woman's symbolic union with her inner masculine dimension, while the blue zone guides this union to create a divine child—a new emergence of an inner potential that must now be nurtured by the maternal aspects of the psyche.

The Buddhist Third Way

The Buddhists describe the Healing Zone as the Third Way. When you reach a river, the safest place is on either side, but staying put gets you nowhere. The most turbulent place is the flowing current in the middle of the river. When you risk this third possibility, you may be swept away, but you are also more likely to reach your destination—the ocean, the spiritual source and destination of all existence. Jung's work and clinical methods provide a guide for engaging this flow and finding your own center of value and purpose in this life. Specifically, he evolved the clinical method of active imagination to engage this flow—the middle way between the ego and the soul. In your daily life, you must always struggle to stay in your body with your instincts. At the same time, you must remain reflective, with the guidance of your soul to help you navigate the middle way. Christ did not just have lofty spiritual ideas; he actually put his life on the line and sacrificed his body on the cross to fulfill his spiritual destiny as Savior. The Holy Spirit guided his values. In the end, he chose spiritual purpose over the survival instinct.

Our lives are a constant dance between instinct and Spirit, pulling us in opposite directions in a struggle between the animal nature of our reptilian brains and the rationality enthroned in our neocortical brains (Rosen, 2003). When this struggle pulls us in contrary directions, the limbic brain and its archetypes offer an image or symbol to unite these opposites—the *Uroboros*, or tail-eating serpent. The Uroboros is a connecting symbol for the triune brain and a manifestation of wholeness. The center of this serpent is the soul, which creates the Healing Zone to organize your instincts and spiritual purpose into a meaningful circle (mandala) that activates healing. The Uroboros symbolizes the idea that your life should not meander like a snake on the prowl for a victim, but should become one with its instinctual tail to gain a spiritual, reflective trajectory.

The Uroboros embodies the gap, the flow, between instinct and Spirit—between the body and the soul, between matter and the psyche. What connects these dots is the fourth dimension of consciousness—Jung's psychoid space and Buddha's Third Way. This dimension is invisible, but remains accessible to consciousness through archetypes, which we will discuss in the next chapter.

In Jungian analytical psychology, we see further evidence of this unity in the phenomena of synchronicity and transcendent function. When struggling with real-life dilemmas, your psyche offers you transcendent functions—dreams, symbols, symptoms, and images—to guide you to your soul's prescription for your maladies. In medical school, I found myself uncertain about my future with the woman I was dating because of the sharp edge to her personality, so I decided to call off the relationship. However, the night before my planned last dinner with her, I dreamed she gave me a pretty red rose with a small thorn on its stem. The dream image guided me out of my ambivalence. I decided to propose to her and am writing this paragraph on the thirty-sixth anniversary of our wedding!

Synchronicity is another way your psyche guides you toward unity. Perhaps you are involved in an internal debate over whether to call a long-lost friend or allow the relationship to lapse. The universe may decide for you with a synchronistic event—the friend you are thinking of calls after twenty years of silence.

The Healing Zone puts you in an elastic transitional state where matter and psyche, past and present, present and future, cause and effect, distance and proximity, temporality and timelessness, instinct and Spirit exist in a seamless, interchangeable continuum. As human observers, we create concepts like time and space, past and future, to help us comprehend the material universe around us. When you use these constructs of the psyche to observe and comprehend the universe, you are essentially observing your own psyche. This positions you to transcend yourself in the fourth transitional state of consciousness and reconnect with the universe as it is. This "universe as it is" is what Jung calls the collective or objective consciousness and what the Hindus call the Primal Spirit or Brahmana—the unrepresentable archetypal psyche identical in all individuals and cultures. You recognize these archetypes in your life because they activate a strong feeling around a certain event or person. For example, when a man views a beautiful woman who is a nurse or physician, the affect depends on the archetype mediating his perception of her. If he is seriously ill, she is perceived through the archetype of Savior or Healer as kind and maternal. In this context, the archetype of the Great Mother mediates the perception. If a man meets that same woman in a social context, he may see her as an object of Eros, with the archetype of the Lover mediating the perception. There is no absolute reality, only subjective reality. We see what we seek unconsciously.

Jung summarizes his wisdom on the Healing Zone in his unfinished masterwork, *Mysterium Coniunctionis* (1970). Jung was trying to establish the interconnection between different manifestations of the mind in our nature, our emotions, our cognition, our spirituality, our bodies, and the world (see figure 3). His formulation has significant clinical and practical implications for understanding and healing human suffering. If an unresolved relationship issue is not resolved, the resulting stress may cause heart problems. Similarly, an unmodulated sexual drive may lead to prostate cancer.

The gold of this hypothesis lies in its treatment implications. If a problem in one realm can be traced to its origins, the mind can be reset from illness to wellness. Quantum physics is extremely applicable here. By activating the Healing Zone, we enter a transcendent realm where emotions, thoughts, and physical and mental symptoms can be reset from disease to health. Unless healers are looking for these connections and trust that they can enter this Healing

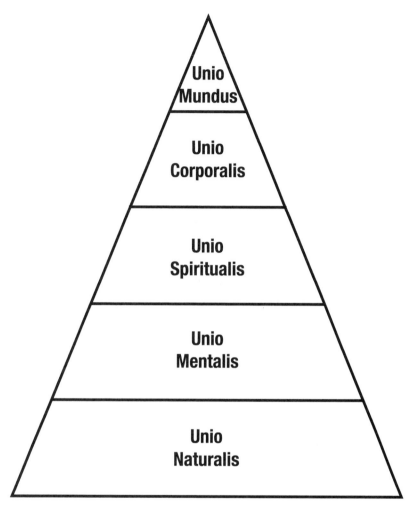

Figure 3. Mysterium coniuntionis.

Zone, the way will not become apparent either to them or to their patients. This is the path of alchemy.

When I discussed this hypothesis with my wife, my analogy was one of a distorted face on a computer screen. Correcting the binary code in the computer program can reset the image. She retorted that it is one thing to reset an image on a computer screen and quite another to correct a facial problem in real life. My response was that sometimes we can. If a person's facial distortion is related to a genetic disorder, we may be getting close to the day when a genomic reset in the patient's DNA can actually help reconfigure parts of the body and the mind. An understanding of genetics and/ or quantum physics provides the two missing pieces of the puzzle that kept Jung from developing his *Mysterium Coniunctionis* to the fullest potential of its therapeutic implications. It is a task we must now pursue.

In *Mysterium Coniunctionis*, Jung lays the foundation for modern mind/body medicine and points to future directions in medical science. Recent developments like neuroimaging and technologies that study the impact of learning and memory at the synaptic level have helped to complete the picture Jung began to sketch. According to the *Mysterium*, there are five steps to crossing the Healing Zone. The first is to acknowledge your authentic nature. A lion does not eat grass and a lamb does not go hunting. You must begin by understanding and accepting your authentic nature. As the saying goes: "Unto thine own self be true."

The second step is to examine the confusing aspects of your psyche; study its components and lay out a map of your personality, including its light and shadow aspects, its superior and inferior abilities, and its perception of your inner masculine (*animus*) or inner feminine (*anima*).

The third step is to understand your personality and life in the context of your spiritual purpose and calling. For a long time, I thought this was the highest purpose and goal of soul work. As a Hindu, the idea of a *dharmic,* or spiritual, purpose and its conscious recognition was appealing to me. However, thanks to Jung, I came to appreciate that this is not the final destination, only an intermediate stage.

The fourth and crucial step in the *magnum opus* of your life journey is to live out these insights into your authentic nature through the body. In other words, you must put your body and life on the line for your spiritual purpose and in accord with your own personality or nature. These insights must be brought to life with the help of your physical body, which now becomes a *yantra*— an instrument of the divine and its instruction. This is the highest union and alchemical alignment with your different states of consciousness. Moses did not just write about his insights; he chose exile from a princely life and wandered for forty years to guide his people. Jesus Christ did not seek political office or power, but surrendered his body to the cross to redeem his children out of love and forgiveness. Gautama Buddha did not just establish schools, universities, and hospitals to heal the suffering; he put his body on the line and lived a monastic life to guide his fellow human beings through compassion.

The Healing Zone of consciousness is analogous to the biblical image of the transfiguration of Jesus. As reported in the Synoptic Gospels, Jesus is transfigured upon a mountain (Matthew 17:1–9, Mark 9:2–8, Luke 9:28–36). He becomes radiant, speaks with Moses and Elijah (preeminent figures in Judaism), and is called "Son" by God. The event was witnessed by three of his closest disciples. In analytical terms, this transfiguration symbolizes present consciousness informed by the archetypal wisdom represented by Moses and Elijah and blessed by God and the healing wisdom of the universe to achieve a higher consciousness. Transfiguration is the holding of consciousness that assimilates the old archetypal wisdom on a given matter at hand. This—experienced by the ego of the individual, witnessed by the therapist, guru, or mentor, and blessed by God or the healing wisdom of the universe—creates a new consciousness that is represented by Christ, Krishna, Buddha, or other symbols of the soul in different traditions.

One of my patients had a crisis at work involving conflict with a supervisor and was nearly fired. He was in the right, but was politically outmaneuvered. He diplomatically backed off, but remained unsure of how to respond to similar crises in the future. Then he had the following dream. He was at a large outdoor service at the top of a mountain, with a stream flowing nearby. There were lots of people in the water with a human skeleton. He felt that the water signified baptism. The skeleton in the water represented his old complexes, which impacted his relationship with authority figures and often got him into trouble. For him, the mountain represented his own Mount of Transfiguration where he received insight about his problem, as witnessed by his analyst. Here, he was informed by the archetypal wisdom of the Trickster about what he needed to do to navigate his turbulent workplace and life. Here, he received God's blessing to follow a new spiritual trajectory in his life and work. In this new consciousness, he had to sacrifice his ego's pride and attend to the task at hand in ways that would serve the universe.

This dream prompted my patient to modify his ways. By integrating humility, acceptance, and diplomacy, he focused on his mission rather than on political victories. He learned to be prepared to lose his ego battles in order to win the war and serve God.

From Stress to Relaxation

Real or perceived threats activate your sympathetic nervous system. When you are in a safe environment, the activity in the hypothalamus—the region of the brain governing sleep cycles and body temperature—is usually minimal. If a new stimulus, even a loud noise, is perceived as a potential danger, a signal is relayed from the sensory cortex of the brain through the hypothalamus—which regulates the body's balance—to the brain stem or the reptilian brain. As a result, you become alert and attentive to your environment. This is called the "initial adaptive vigilance response."

If the danger level rises from potential to immediate, your body responds with a more intense and prolonged discharge from the hypothalamus, activating the sympathetic division of the reptilian nervous system through the release of adrenaline from the adrenal glands (see figure 4). Symptoms of this acute stress response

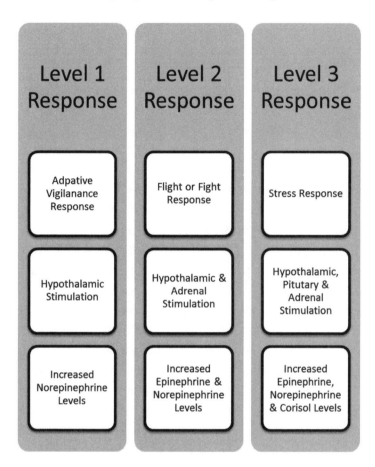

Figure 4. The stress response.

include an acceleration of heartbeat and breathing, inhibition of the stomach and intestines, constriction of blood vessels in many parts of the body, dilation of blood vessels for muscles, inhibition of the lachryal gland responsible for tears and saliva, dilation of the pupils, relaxation of the bladder, inhibition of erections, hearing loss or loss of peripheral vision, and the subjective experience of fear, anxiety, and panic.

The manifestations of acute stress prepare you for fighting, fleeing, or freezing. If stress continues unabated, your physical body exhibits a full-spectrum response involving the hypothalamus and the pituitary and adrenal glands, as well as the sympathetic nervous system and the endocrine system. As a result, the sympathetic nervous system pumps stress-managing chemicals into your body and a major stress hormone into your blood, bringing your body, brain, and endocrine system to a knife-sharp response to the situation. The interactions among these organs constitute the hypothalamic pituitary adrenal (HPA) axis, the part of the neuroendocrine system that controls reactions to stress and regulates many body processes, including digestion, the immune system, moods and emotions, sexuality, and your metabolic or energy-management system.

The hypothalamus contains neurons that synthesize and secrete vasopressin and corticotrophin-releasing hormone (CRH), triggering the production of cortisol, a major stress hormone that affects many tissues in the body, including the brain. Cortisol has many important functions, including modulation of stress reactions. An excess of cortisol, however, can be damaging to the hippocampus of the brain. Deficiencies of the hippocampus may reduce the memory resources that help the body respond appropriately to stress. High cortisol levels as a result of chronic stress compromise the immune system, which in turn leads to higher rates of infection and long-term immune-system disorder. Eventually, however, the adrenal glands may be overwhelmed, resulting in feeble or inadequate production of cortisol.

Most Western medical treatments for stress-related illnesses—anxiety, depression, and post-traumatic-stress disorders—work by activating the sympathetic nervous system and increasing the brain's neurotransmitter levels of serotonin, norepinephrine, and dopamine. While these put out the fire of the symptoms of stress, the cost of using up the body's emergency reserves compromises health in the long run. Western medicine stamps out the fire, but fails to plug the "gas leak" in the system that caused it. It never addresses the root cause of stress. This gap can be filled by Eastern healing methods, which stimulate the soothing and healing parasympathetic nervous system by activating the Healing Zone.

Adrenal Fatigue

Chronic stress overwhelms the adrenal glands and leads to clinical states of depression, fibromyalgia, and chronic fatigue syndromes. In holistic and alternative medicine, this adrenal overload is referred to as adrenal fatigue (see figure 5).

According to Mayo Clinic endocrinologist Todd B. Nippoldt, adrenal fatigue is a term for a collection of symptoms, including body aches, fatigue, nervousness, sleep disturbances, and digestive problems (Nippoldt, 2011). While he feels that it is not an accepted medical diagnosis, in my clinical experience, it is often a good template for understanding a patient's response to chronic stress. According to Nippoldt, the adrenal glands produce a variety of hormones that are essential to life. The medical term "adrenal insufficiency," or Addison's disease, refers to inadequate production of one or more of these hormones as a result of an underlying disease. Signs and symptoms of adrenal insufficiency include fatigue, body aches, unexplained weight loss, low blood pressure, lightheadedness, and loss of body hair. Adrenal insufficiency can be diagnosed by blood tests and special stimulation tests that show inadequate levels of adrenal hormones.

Proponents of the adrenal fatigue diagnosis claim that it is a mild form of adrenal insufficiency caused by chronic stress. The unproven theory behind adrenal fatigue is that your adrenal glands are unable to keep pace with the demands of perpetual fight-or-flight-or-freeze arousal. As a result, they can't produce quite enough of the hormones you need to feel well. Existing blood tests, according to this theory, aren't sensitive enough to detect such a small decline in adrenal function—but your body is. That's why you feel tired, weak, and depressed.

Conventional endocrinology tests cannot diagnose adrenal fatigue, because they register only extreme dysfunction in the adrenals—for example, Addison's disease, a potentially fatal condition in which the adrenals essentially shut down. Holistic or complementary practitioners diagnose more subtle dysfunctions in your adrenal glands with a saliva cortisol test. While this controversy over the medical acceptance of the diagnosis of adrenal fatigue syndrome is interesting from an academic perspective, most of us are painfully aware of the impact of chronic stress on our adrenal systems.

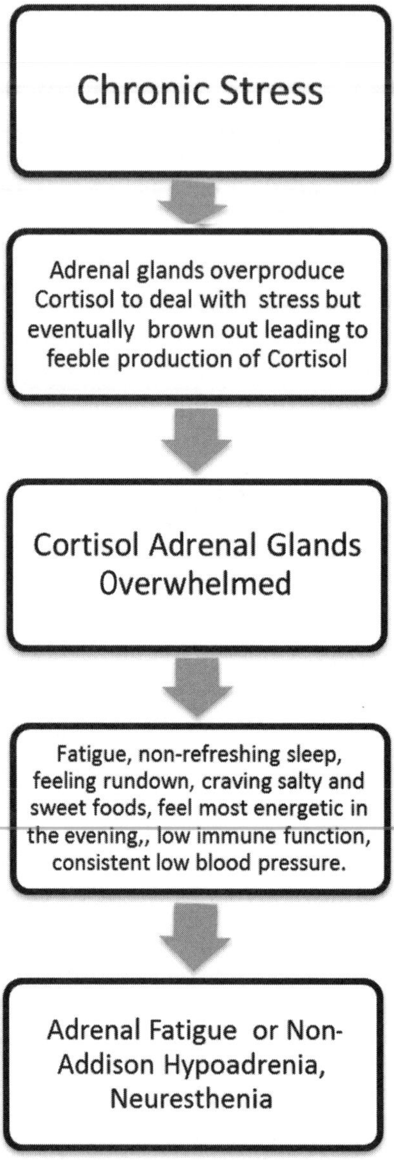

The Relaxation Response

Eastern healing and meditative practices activate the relaxation response of the body in the fourth state of consciousness, the Healing Zone (see figure 6). This fourth state has a calming, cooling, soothing, restorative, healing influence on the brain and the body through the parasympathetic nervous system. It lowers blood pressure and oxygen consumption, reduces respiratory and heart rates, alleviates muscle tension, and increases alpha waves, enabling us to achieve a sacred state of mindfulness (Srinivasan, 2006).

Chronic Stress

Adrenal glands overproduce Cortisol to deal with stress but eventually brown out leading to feeble production of Cortisol

Cortisol Adrenal Glands Overwhelmed

Fatigue, non-refreshing sleep, feeling rundown, craving salty and sweet foods, feel most energetic in the evening,, low immune function, consistent low blood pressure.

Adrenal Fatigue or Non-Addison Hypoadrenia, Neuresthenia

Figure 5. Adrenal fatigue syndrome.

It is probable that the relaxation response (Benson, 1975) of mind and body is mediated primarily by acetylcholine and secondarily by the attachment hormone oxytocin. Other neurotransmitter systems, like gamma amino butyric acid (GABA) inhibition, may play an additional role in restoring parasympathetic activity in the nervous system. The role of the parasympathetic nervous system is crucial for psychiatrists to be able to understand and treat numerous disorders triggered by an imbalance between the sympathetic and parasympathetic systems. This understanding, the foundation of the Eastern healing paradigm, has not been readily acknowledged by Western physicians, but is gradually entering the outer precincts of medical science. For example, in treating severe depression after even electro-shock therapy has failed, some physicians try to stimulate the vagus nerve, which increases parasympathetic activity, to restore a calm, serene mental state. To stimulate the vagus nerve, a device called a pulse generator is surgically implanted in the chest and a wire threaded under the skin that connects the pulse generator to the left vagus nerve in the neck. The pulse generator sends out electrical signals along the nerve to the brain. These signals affect mood centers in the brain, possibly improving depression symptoms (Burke, 2006; Sackeim, 2006).

It is possible to harvest the benefits of parasympathetic activation without surgical implants, however, by accessing the Healing Zone through ancient treatment rituals, including pranayama, meditation, mindfulness, centering prayer, relaxation training, and yoga.

On a scale of 1 to 10, our initial, instinctive response to stress usually soars to Level 10, the maximum response, through a reflexive reaction in the sympathetic nervous system. This occurs without any modulation by the limbic or neocortical brain. When we are at Level 10, we are bereft, not only of reason, but also of the archetypal wisdom of our ancestors.

Alternatively, trauma victims who have been beaten down

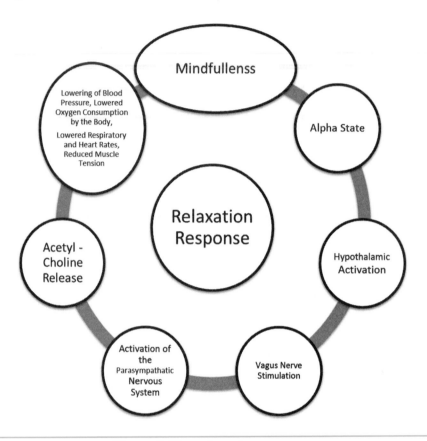

Figure 6. The relaxation response.

emotionally and burned out by repeated, wounding experiences can dissociate from the causes of their stress. Their response to real danger may be dangerously limited or they may have no response at all. This is a Level 1 response.

Both ends of this scale are maladaptive. The Level 10 response is a reaction of fight-or-flight without temperance, discernment, or consciousness (Cannon, 1915). The Level 1 response is disengaged from real danger and has the potential to re-traumatize and jeopardize the well-being and safety of the individual. Over three decades of clinical experience, I have found that the optimal response is a

Level 5 response—a measured, reflective, thoughtful, proportionate response to the external or internal threat or danger. A sober and soulful Level 5 response comes from assessing the danger or situation using the nervous system's capacity for cognitive reasoning, and adding the archetypal and ancestral wisdom of the nervous system. It is a calm, centered, coordinated, whole-body response that engages with the parasympathetic nervous system. Level 5 responses may not be dramatic, but they are measured, proportionate, and adaptive. They factor in a realistic assessment of danger and bring to bear the totality of the individual's potential to form an adequate response. They bring into play, not only the personal consciousness, but also ancestral, archetypal wisdom.

I have seen this vividly demonstrated in patients who are recovering from addiction. In dealing with stressful situations, they instinctively go to Level 10. For them, this response maximizes and "catastrophizes" any potential danger, prompting drug cravings as a way to soothe and calm themselves. This leads to abuse of drugs, alcohol, food, sex, and gambling to modulate the stress. The management of cravings, which calls for moving down from Level 10 to Level 5 responses, has become a focus in the recovery process for addicts.

When an individual undergoes a Level 10 response to a given situation or stressor and feels overwhelmed by feelings of fear, anger, sadness, excessive happiness, shame, or guilt, this can be a precursor to a drug or addictive craving. I counsel my patients to activate a cravings-management protocol immediately (see below). The first step in this is for them to recognize that they are having a craving. Next, I advise them to identify the trigger event and to appraise it consciously. I have found that addicts and individuals struggling with depression or anxiety often have a faulty, warped cognitive lens through which they appraise themselves and others, and situations. Cognitive therapists from Aaron Beck's school of psychology refer to this as a cognitive distortion, which often comes down to black-or-white thinking, all-or-none thinking, using

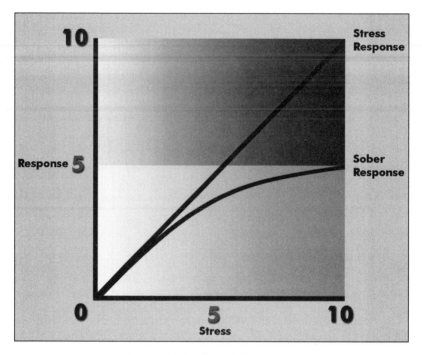

Figure 7. The Level 5 response.

boiler-plate "should" criteria to judge themselves, events, and the world, or personalizing, catastrophizing, or minimizing situations. These cognitive distortions result in feelings of fear, anger, sadness, shame, and guilt that are far more exaggerated than reality calls for. The body then jumps to a Level 10 response, made battle-ready by a maladaptive flight-or-flight reaction to the situation. At Level 10, a person may resort to the nuclear option to swat a fly!

The goal of recovery management is to reappraise stressful situations without resorting to reflexive, distorted, automatic thoughts. This reappraisal leads to a more realistic assessment of the situation and a measured, proportionate, sober, and adaptive response that averts cravings and a relapse into addiction. The paradigm is summarized in figure 7.

Cravings-Management Plan

- Recognize that you have a craving.
- Identify the event that triggered the craving.
- Assess the cognitive distortion associated with the craving.
- Identify how you feel about the craving—anger, sadness, joy, fear, guilt, or shame.
- Rate the strength of the feeling on scale of 1 to 10 (1 is minimum; 10 is maximum).
- Explore a sober or rational alternative explanation for the trigger event.
- Acknowledge a sober thought and feeling consistent with a more rational, alternative explanation for the trigger event.
- Decide what you can and cannot do about the event.
- Do what you can in the next twenty-four hours and turn the rest over to the healing wisdom of the universe.
- Center yourself by prayer, meditation, music, journaling, yoga, pranayama, reading, calling a friend, or attending a meeting.

Now that we have explored the mystery and the science of the Healing Zone, we will investigate the timeless myths and archetypes that guide us through this Zone from illness to wellness.

Chapter 2

Archetypes—Your Guides through the Healing Zone

In your life journey through the Healing Zone, archetypes can help you navigate the flow from illness to wellness. Archetypes are defined in Jungian literature as the cumulative wisdom of the human mind activated in each person to help us through our spiritual development and achieve wellness. Transmitted genetically, these archetypes are mediated by the nervous system and by our formative development. The archetypal patterns are the natural laws or "dynamic skeletons" that structure our expectations and our experiences. When an archetype is activated, the instructions in it organize what we see, how we feel, the way we depict our experiences, and what we do with them. This process is independent of conscious choice and we are unaware of it operating in the background.

Archetypes have crystallized over millions of years of human experience (Stevens, 2005) and are the default modes of our unconscious adaptation. They are activated to deal with important life events and changes like birth, death, marriage, leaving home, illness and recovery, crisis, and trauma. It is the task of your consciousness to modify these default templates in ways that are consistent with your personal attributes and circumstances. In the course of development, you fill out and reanimate the vestiges of the experiences of your ancestors.

Given an appropriate stimulus, your psyche activates the corresponding archetype to respond optimally and adapt to the situation at hand. However, archetypes have a tendency to provoke projections. For instance, if you are caught in the Mother archetype, you may project the unconscious image and expectations of your mother onto another individual. You may start behaving with your boss, spouse, or therapist as if that person were your mother. The projection may not always be appropriate.

Robert was in therapy for symptoms of depression and excessive involvement in work, to the detriment of his marriage and his relationship with his daughters. He was unable to relax or play. Robert was caught in the Hero archetype. He felt like a great warrior who had to win every corporate battle. His story revealed that he had had an alcoholic father and a depressed mother. The only way Robert could survive emotionally, protect his younger siblings, and receive affirmation was by heroic successes. This is a familiar adaptation in the adult children of alcoholics.

Gradually, Robert understood his personal myth of a hero-warrior, and began to balance work with love, play, creativity, and spirituality. Nevertheless, he continued to struggle with residual depression unless he overachieved at work. We agreed that, rather than fight the Hero archetype, he must honor it. As a result, Robert began to devote his professional energy to improving the welfare of his employees and local community. When he balanced his professional energy between success and service, Robert's depression was much improved. The Hero archetype ultimately guided his journey from illness to wellness.

The archetypes that guide you in the Healing Zone have a quality of bringing two states of consciousness into alignment so that a new state emerges that restores health and wholeness—although the archetypes may not always seem to offer a rational response to your life crises. When Mahatma Gandhi repaid British aggression with love and compassion, his apparently irrational response was in reality a profound answer coming out of the Guru/Guide archetype. When you receive archetypal guidance through your dreams, your creative output, your complexes, your medical and psychiatric problems, or your relationship tangles, or through synchronistic events and accidents or myths and fairy tales, you must suspend judgment and honor them in your life.

Let's explore the five archetypes that help us in our transit through the Healing Zone from illness to wellness. Each of these myths has specific prescriptions for healing, which are given at the end of each section.

The Lion Man

In the Hindu scriptures, Vishnu is charged with maintaining cosmic order; he incarnates in our world to restore spiritual order. These incarnations are called *avatars*. The same phenomenon occurs in your individual consciousness. When your life gets off track, an archetypal activation of the deeper wisdom of your soul guides your ego, or outer consciousness, back from illness to wellness.

In Hindu mythology, Vishnu is incarnated as Narasimha, the Lion Man, to destroy the king of demons, who retired to the mountain and began *tapas*, a form of meditation and penance, pleasing the gods with his devotion (see figure 8). Brahma appeared to the demon king and said: "Arise. I have never seen such a devoted meditation before. Ask for whatever you desire." The demon replied: "Great Lord, if you will grant my prayer, this is what I seek: Let not death come to me from any creature created by you; let me not meet with death either in the house or outside it; let not my death occur either during the day or at night; no man-made weapon should cause my death; I should not die either on land, sea, or in the sky."

After receiving this blessing, the demon exceeded all bounds of oppression and dethroned Indra, the king of the heavens. All the gods were filled with fear. Indra, along with the other gods, appeared before Brahma and prayed for deliverance. Brahma said that he could not undo his blessing, but advised Indra to go to Vishnu for assistance. Vishnu promised to destroy the demon king in due course.

The demon king had a son named Prahalad, who was a devotee

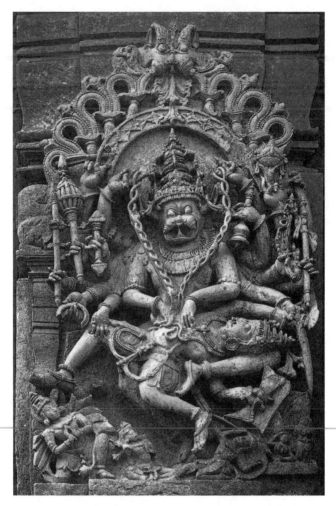

Figure 8. The Lion Man, archetype of the
fourth dimension of consciousness.

of Vishnu and protested his father's demonic ways. The king tried to destroy his son in a fit of anger. He tied a stone to Prahalad's body and threw him into the river, but Vishnu rescued him from drowning. The king later tried to have his son trampled under the feet of an elephant, but the elephant lifted Prahalad lovingly by its trunk and put him on its back. The king then built a house for Prahalad and set it on fire, but even this could not harm him. The father tried to poison the son, but to no avail.

At last, the king thundered at the boy: "You are a disgrace to your family. You have betrayed me. You have been led astray. Reveal to me who has influenced you against me." The earth trembled as the king roared at the boy, but the prince calmly replied: "Dear father, it was Vishnu who gave me this courage. He is stronger than you, I, the universe; even Brahma is humbled by his strength. He is the Protector of the Universe."

The mighty demon king held all the gods under his thumb, yet a mere child challenged his authority. The king, mad with rage and no longer able to control himself, tried to kill the prince with his sword. At that very moment, Vishnu appeared in the form of the Lion Man, caught the demon king with a loud roar, and carried him to the threshold of the hall. He sat on the threshold with the demon in his lap. Then he dug his claws deep into the king's body and tore it open. Narasimha, the Lion Man, finally killed the demon.

Vishnu, in the person of the Lion Man, killed the demon at dusk, which is neither day nor night. He killed him at the threshold, a place that is neither outside the house nor inside in it. The king was killed in the lap of the god, which is neither sea, nor land, nor sky. He was not killed by any weapons, but torn by the claws of the Lion Man. He was not killed by anyone created by Brahma, but rather by Vishnu, from whose navel Brahma was created.

Prescription of the Lion Man Archetype

This story is very instructive for our purposes.

- Whenever your life gets out of spiritual order and your ego (the demon king) takes charge, it is time for the Vishnu archetype to incarnate to reset your path. The Narasimha avatar is the prototype of the fourth dimension of consciousness, which is essential in creating a new consciousness to guide your path.

- The fourth dimension is neither awake nor asleep; it is at the threshold of wakefulness and sleep, deep sleep, and dreaming. In this state, you are not in your human or animal nature, but in your soul or universal consciousness. You are not on land (awake) or sea (asleep) or in the sky (dream consciousness).
- It not the king or the ego that can summon this energy; it is the demon's son who summons Vishnu for help. In psychological terms, this means that the humbler, marginalized aspects of your personality are what usher in new beginnings and change. For example, if you are extroverted, solitude and introversion can connect you to your soul. If you are a logical, thinking individual, it is your neglected but subtle feelings that point the way to solving life's problems.
- Often, when you refuse to tame your narcissism, it is your loved ones, your spouse, or your children who verbalize the protest of your soul. In this myth, the demon king symbolizes your ego infected by narcissism or complexes. When your ego gets out of sync with your soul, you can be aided by the archetype of the Vishnu avatar to destroy your demon king—the old ego adaptation, the "business-as-usual" scenario—and make room for the prince, or a fresh and new adaptation.
- The fourth dimension of consciousness is a crucial bridge to this archetypal energy. This story can help you understand the unique properties of this consciousness. It teaches you how to recognize it when you encounter it, and how to invoke and honor it.

Aditi

One of the most significant obstacles to engaging your full potential is your discomfort with the dynamics of the void. We are generally fearful of the void, but if you can hold the tension between the void and clutter, you can tune in to the Healing Zone. The great rishis, the holy men and women of the East, have long postulated that we live in three states of consciousness: wakefulness, sleep, and dreaming. But the transition between these states involves engaging the gap between them. In this gap, you are tuned in to the flow of the great energies of the universe, its timeless wisdom, its infinite void, its immense potential for new creation, and its countless possibilities.

The void is also a realm of great danger, however, where the uninitiated can get lost in the dark side of the cosmos and never find their way back into human consciousness. Different meditative traditions from all the great cultures have developed guidelines for engaging this sacred space in a soulful way. Transcendental meditation is one such tradition. The archetype of Aditi guides you in this realm—the gap, the flow, the void—and paves the way for you to tap into the vast potential of the wisdom of the universe (see figure 9).

Aditi symbolizes the energy of the void, the sacred space that is essential to engaging the Healing Zone. Our tendency is to fill in the void with clutter rather than honoring and nurturing it. If you are sitting quietly in the evening, perhaps you just can't resist turning on the television rather than reflecting and meditating. When you are driving your car, you may flip on the radio rather than permitting yourself time to muse. When you are walking, perhaps you put on headphones rather than tune in to the nature around you. We rarely allow the void to whisper to us. If only you can resist trampling the void, however, Aditi may speak to you from the depths of your soul and inspire you with a creative new fantasy, image, thought, impulse, or possibility that can set in motion the incarnation of a new consciousness in your routine life. Whenever I have resisted the temptations of outer distractions and honored the sacred void, the inspiring and healing guidance of Aditi has blessed me. This has permitted my patients and me to make new beginnings on our paths from illness to wellness.

Perhaps the most outstanding attribute of Aditi is her motherhood. As a mothering presence, Aditi is often asked to guard those who petition her. Appropriate to her role as a mother, Aditi is sometimes associated with a cow. As an earthly cow, she provides nourishment; as a cosmic cow, her milk is identified with the redemptive, renewing mythic elixir of the gods.

Aditi is often experienced as a new creative impulse just at the moment when you are exhausted and preoccupied with outer life. Jungian psychoanalyst Marie-Louise Von Franz describes this as a "Spiritus Creator" in the unconscious that manifests as a creative impulse and stirs up new possibilities (Von Franz 2001).

I once worked with a schizophrenic who fiddled with his fingers throughout our therapy sessions. Later, he admitted to an obsession with knives; he had a large collection at home. On his way to my office, he often picked up pieces of wood from tree branches and fiddled with these twigs. Prior to one of our sessions, it occurred to me that my patient should try to do something creative with his fingers, knives, and twigs. After a conference in Boston, where I had bought a small scrimshaw engraving on a nut palm, I suggested that he try whittling. Soon he started to make beautiful whittled images out of wooden branches and his anxiety was much reduced. I was even able to reduce his dose of psychotropic medications. I was still curious, however, about his whittling, knives, and finger-fidgeting rituals. I dug deeper into his family history and, to my surprise, learned that one of his great-grandfathers was a member of the American whaling fleet. Scrimshaw is the traditional art form of American whalers, who fashioned jewelry and other articles from whale ivory while at sea.

At other times, Aditi manifests in the psychoid space, where archetypes crystallize as attitudes, drives, complexes, apparently chance events, moods, and physical and psychological symptoms. These experiences are not only psychological; they are also physical and may evoke synchronistic phenomena. When you experience a synchronistic event, Aditi may be whispering to you.

The manifestations of Aditi may take several psychological forms. When you are in her realm, your psyche is in a state of void,

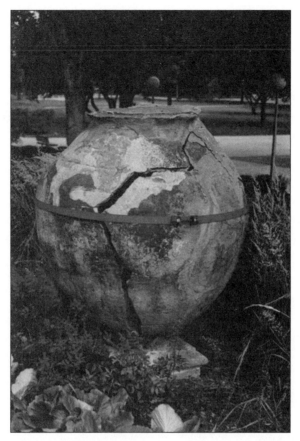

Figure 9. Aditi, patron goddess of the Healing Zone
(Marquette University—Milwaukee, Wisconsin)

or emptiness. If you don't confuse this with depression or pathology and hold the energy of the void for long enough, your unconscious steps in and activates the archetype of Aditi, allowing it to manifest itself in the creation of new consciousness, often through mythic, folkloric, or fairytale figures. A big intuition may manifest as a giant; a small inkling may manifest as a dwarf. Sometimes, these may manifest as extraterrestrials, which signifies an intuition completely outside of the realm of your consciousness. When honored, these manifestations may lead to an expansion of ego consciousness.

When human reason has reached its limits in discerning the message of Aditi, your feeling function zeros in on the promptings of the goddess. In any given enterprise, when you have followed your hunches, examined all the details, and thought through all the logical options, yet are still uncertain about the path, it is your feeling—your assessment of what you value most in the situation—that guides your final decision. It is your heart—your feeling function—that is the final arbiter of your most crucial choices.

When I migrated from the UK to the United States, I did extensive research about where I would settle. My gut feeling was California, where intuition said that my Eastern background might be better understood. My assessment of details suggested the Mayo Clinic as the place where I could flourish professionally. My logical assessment pointed to Chicago, where I could pursue my academic goals. But my heart called me to the solitude and peacefulness of Milwaukee. It was a good choice. Milwaukee has permitted me to do my work of integrating Eastern and Western wisdom in a relatively quiet space, uncluttered by other pressures and influences. This choice was the gift of Aditi.

Another patient of mine, Virgo, is good example of how feelings can eventually redeem your soul under the auspices of Aditi. Virgo is a very logical man, attentive to detail—traits that served him well as a physician. His Waterloo was in the realm of feelings. After a turbulent divorce, he started dating his present wife. He was uncertain of this emerging relationship and skeptical of his capacity to make any new relationship work. Then he had the following dream, which helped him with his dilemma.

He and his wife are living aboard an old rusty ship, possibly an old oil tanker no longer in use. They make love. An unknown person or persons disturb them—perhaps even attack them. He looks out the old, rusty, loose-fitting door, but there is no one there. They have a daughter, a little girl who is about six or seven years old. She has been taking violin lessons. He hasn't heard her play for a while, and he asks her to play. She plays a beautiful piece that has lots of underlying fine rhythmic fabric with a melody overlaying it. He is very impressed with her ability and proud of her. He shuffles around in bed, half awake. His wife wakes him up and he gets up and ponders the dream.

Virgo's ambivalence about marrying Jenny, which was rooted in the burn-out he felt from his first marriage, was represented by the rusty old oil tanker. Maybe the vessel needed restoration. I was the unknown intruder, the therapist Virgo felt was critical of his marriage plans. Actually, this was a projection of his own ambivalence about the relationship. The little girl symbolized his *anima,* or feeling function. He took piano lessons at age six to seven and his mother played piano.

The dream was a positive sign. The violin symbolized further amplification of his feeling function—the music of the soul. Jenny evoked feelings of love, desire, passion, and value, but—most important—touched the violin strings of his heart and soul. The dream was blessing his emerging relationship with Jenny. Aditi had blessed their union.

In number symbolism, the number three indicates the presence of Aditi and signifies the creative flow. Four indicates the number of differentiated consciousness (the four functions, the four directions, the four seasons), in which the creative thrust of the number three has been assimilated into emerging consciousness. Four results from the flow of three and becomes still, visible, and ordered within ego consciousness.

To put it another way, Aditi gets you into the void of consciousness, paving the way for your descent into the unconscious in search of new symbols for personal growth. When you have three quarters of the pie, you delve into your soul depths to look for the missing fourth piece, where the answer to the riddle usually lies. It is the three that leaves a sense of unfinished assessment and provokes the search for the fourth dimension. The fourth dimension then incarnates the creation myth of the individual, most apparent in your initial or big dreams.

Jung (1982)) attached special significance to initial dreams in the therapeutic process. He postulated that the dreams that appear in the initial stages of analysis often bring to light the essential root cause of problems and also hold the key with which to unlock the path to the soul. Jung observed that initial dreams are often amazingly lucid and clear-cut. As the work of analysis progresses, however, dreams tend to lose their clarity. It seems that initial dreams provide individuals with the best possible glimpse of the unconscious, and provide a map of the personal myths that guide them to initiate new beginnings. As an analogy, we can see that the best view of the sun is at sunrise as it dramatically crests the eastern horizon out of the darkness of the night (the unconscious). But as the day progresses, the sun's orb blends into the glare and glitter of daylight and the clarity that comes from the juxtaposition of day and night—the past and the future, the conscious and the unconscious—is lost.

Initial dreams are a unique window into the mystery of the soul under the auspices of the Aditi archetype. Whenever there is a feeling of void in your personal life, when your ego consciousness has reached its limit in the management of a problem in your outer or inner life, Aditi presides over the psychic situation to guide you. She gifts your consciousness with a dream, a synchronistic event, an image, a fantasy, or an inspiration that ushers in the creation of new consciousness to help you overcome the crisis at hand. She gives you inspiration for a new beginning.

In the mid-1980s, when I was feeling lost, exiled, and burned-out in Milwaukee, Aditi gifted me with a dream that pointed me to my path. I dreamed that I had a meal with my mentor from India, Father Valles, and two other Jesuit fathers. Later, we prayed together at the college chapel. In my dream, the three fathers were associated with the Christian trinity of Father, Son, and Holy Spirit. Later, I related them to the Hindu trinity of Brahma the Creator, Vishnu the Preserver, and Shiva the Destroyer. Still later, I learned of the goddess consorts, the dynamic energy system that drives these three gods—Saraswati, Laxmi, and Parvati. This dream reset me on my path to integrate Eastern and Western wisdom. It still inspires me and continues to instruct me on the path to my soul in new and novel ways.

John's story is another example of the light of Aditi that guides our way in the darkness of life through the gift of an initial dream. John is a gay professional who sought analysis to deal with his grief about the loss of a relationship with a partner and a lack of passion in life despite considerable professional success. He was in his late thirties, and had a distinct boyish charm. Yet he seemed overburdened by life and outer success, while at the same time disconnected from the care of his body and from attending to his inner life. He grieved over the loss of his partner, a tall, handsome, blonde, blue-eyed model. His ex-partner's new companion was a Latin American man who was the same age as John. In his initial dream, he is at a party and sitting across the room from his ex-boy-friend's table. The ex-boyfriend has not shown up, but his present lover is at the table.

This initial dream was the prescription for John's new begin-ning. As we worked with it in the following weeks, we came to understand that both his ex-boyfriend and his present lover were reflections and fractals of John's own soul. These dream figures could be understood as unconscious manifestations of his soul needing to be assimilated into the wholeness of his personality. The necessary prerequisites for his new beginnings were to honor the void of his present life, the chaos in his relational matrix, the grief over lost love, and the hope for new beginnings. The archetype that ushered in this new beginning was Aditi as she constellated in the session following this dream.

In the session, John reported that he was feeling somewhat sad and tired. It had been a professionally burdened and tiring week. I proposed using guided imagery with this mood to give it form and personhood. His image was of his maternal aunt, Mita, who was a simple soulful woman who never married and who had raised

John's mother and uncles after his grandmother's death. She lived an austere life with few trappings. Upon further analysis, it became apparent that Mita was an *anima* soul figure who had come to guide John in his hour of distress and loss. While his outer life was over-burdened and driven by striving for outer success, his anima, his soul guide, crystallized and led him to a precious image of Mita.

Mita was John's doorway to the void—to the solitude, sim-plicity, and austerity of his soulful life—as a compensation for his success-driven outer life. At the core of the image of Mita was the archetype of Aditi. In John's initial dream, Aditi appeared in an image of void, the empty chair reserved for the missing ex-boy-friend. Incarnated within his blue mood, Aditi appeared as a soul figure granting him a glimpse into a compensatory attitude of a spiritually informed life. The new John had the potential to be more balanced—not only valuing his outer success, but honoring Aditi's call for a reflective life.

Sometimes, our meetings with Aditi come through synchronis-tic events. By the early 1990s, I was burned out by the pressures of managed care and administrative responsibilities at a local psy-chiatric hospital. A brief stint of Freudian training did not feed my soul and I was resigned to life in the clinical trenches. Then, one of my associates, whom I had mistakenly perceived as a professional adversary, decided to move to another part of the country. I saw him as self-aggrandizing and narcissistic. In retrospect, I see that he carried the projection of my dark side. I disliked in him what I now understand as my own unconscious narcissism. However, at his farewell party, my wife and I were seated next to him and his wife. While making small talk with his wife, the conversation turned to dreams. I had just re-read Freud's classic *Interpretation of Dreams* and talked excitedly about my views. She listened attentively and gently said that Carl Jung also had some interesting things to say about dreams. I had minimal familiarity with Jung. In mainstream psychiatric training, we were taught about Jung for less than one hour. The next day, she left Jung's (1984) anthology on dreams as a parting gift in my mailbox.

The book sat on my bookshelf for over a year before I stumbled upon it again when trying to analyze a difficult dream. Suddenly, I was hooked on Jung. This chance event gradually culminated in a deepening interest and eventually formal training in Jungian psychology. It was my apparent adversary's wife who introduced me to my life's calling. The soul whispers in mysterious ways. My brief, but life-changing, encounter with the goddess Aditi occurred during a chance dinner-table conversation.

Individuals who do not recognize and honor their creative impulses can grow obsessed with, even addicted to, various substances or activities in order to divert and drain off their creative drive. Sexual addictions and other addictive behaviors are a particular danger in predisposed individuals. The psychodynamic context of addictive behaviors is a difficulty in holding and honoring the void. In over thirty years of treatment experience with recovering addicts, I have found that, when cravings are traced back to their origins, they are often rooted in a dread of the void and the tendency to replace this feeling quickly with addictive behaviors. Twelve-step recovery programs provide an invaluable service by setting a framework within which to deal with this void through fellowship and spiritual contact with the Higher Power—the great Aditi.

While frantic attempts to flee the void often lead to susceptibility to addictions, succumbing to the void can also result in a host of other psychiatric conditions. These include avoidant, schizoid, and other personality disorders, and, in extreme cases, schizophrenic-spectrum disorders. Preoccupied with the inner world, an individual can shut out the demands of the outer world.

According to Von Franz, creativity is often accompanied by frustration, fear, loneliness, and boredom. When a creative idea crosses the threshold of consciousness and approaches the ego, it attracts libido or psychological energy away from other complexes, hang-ups, or personality traits. The ego consequently feels low, tired, restless, and depressed, until the creative impulse breaks through into consciousness.

The guidance of Aditi has been crucial in my own life. Early in my career, I was an overburdened medical professional, struggling to juggle the competing demands of professional success, parenting my children, maintaining intimacy with my spouse, and surviving as an immigrant in an extremely competitive American environment. In the second half of my life experience, my soul kept tugging at me to connect with my inner life and cultural roots—to make some meaning out of my exile from the land of my origin. The professional and spiritual—the Western and Eastern, the medical and holistic—aspects of my psyche felt *split*. Even in India, my schooling had been carried out under the caring auspices of Jesuit fathers, while my parents were devout Hindus. Between these splits in my psyche resided a sense of void. I was having an Aditi experience.

The Aditi image shown in figure 9 was symbolic of my inner state at the time. I found this rendering of Aditi on the grounds of Marquette, the Jesuit University in Milwaukee. Perhaps the splits in my psyche were ready to heal and I was ready to be whole. Certainly, this image depicted the goddess holding the *broken vessel* of the void in her tight embrace and healing the fissures—perhaps not to perfection, but in a way that encouraged wholeness and unity.

Gradually, Aditi guided me to make room for the Healing Zone. Initially, this involved encountering the void by relinquishing the trappings of external success and professional security. As I started to let go, the void presented me with frightening thoughts and feelings. Would I lose all my patients if I set limits on my work? Would I be a bad father and husband if I did not make a lot of money? As I struggled with these fears, new creative impulses popped up in the form of an interest in depth psychology, Jungian training, photography, and computers. I eventually understood these new interests as gifts of the goddess Aditi. As I gratefully and gradually integrate these new creative structures into my life, I continue to endure the splits within myself under the holding embrace of Aditi. And, of course, my own struggle informs my work with my patients.

Let me share with you story of one of my patients who met and received the guidance of Aditi on his path from illness to wellness.

Often, significant relationships carry fractals of the soul. They become passwords that open the door between the soul and Spirit. This was the case for Edmund, a neurologist who had burned out in his pressure-cooker job. This dissolved his emotional connection with his wife and led to divorce. He entered into a second marriage with a soulful and supportive wife. Although he had the financial resources to retire, he felt that he had no consuming purpose outside of medicine that would sustain his interest. He was fearful of the void of retired life.

In our work together, I immediately had to deal with the deep sense of depression and void Edmund felt in his life. He was unable to decide what to do with himself. As his therapist, I had an intuition that his sense of the void was a significant starting point. It was a sacred place where Aditi had appeared to cleanse him of the *maya* of the past and guide him to his future. We started by ending his habit of drinking in the evening, replacing it with daily walks, journaling for twenty minutes a day, and meditation. As he used these simple devices to honor his void and create sacred space, Aditi gifted him with guidance to create new life structures. He started to attend AA meetings, joined the local medical society, and volunteered to be on a committee to connect with his peers. He started going out on the town twice a week with his wife. Gradually, he focused on the aspects of his practice that he enjoyed the most. Life returned to his practice and relationships. He resumed his interest in flying a small airplane. Out of the void of his depression, Aditi's guidance blessed him with new structures in his life.

In speaking of his children, Edmund reported that his oldest child, Robert, was a model son—a Michigan State graduate like himself and well established as an investment consultant in New York City. His younger son, Stan, was the black sheep of the family. Almost expelled from high school, he had barely finished his undergraduate degree and now worked as a realtor in Las Vegas and enjoyed living the life of a virtual desert bum. On closer analytic reflection, it became clearer that Stan enjoyed Edmund's unlived life. Edmund was overly responsible, while Stan was irresponsible, playful, carefree, social, and spontaneous.

In analysis, Edmund gradually claimed his Stan side—his playful side, the "Stan within." He decided to work in a low-stress environment as a part-time urgent-care physician in an underserved part of Milwaukee, and started to nurture the creative and spiritual sectors of his life. Edmund now feels much more connected with his wife and sons.

I have been amazed to learn how often children carry the unlived projections of their parents' lives, both light and dark. Sometimes, they carry their unlived virtues; at other times, they manifest their unconscious vices. The more conscious you become of your soul, the less you project onto your children and other significant people in your life. You then can live a fuller life and unburden your relationships from having to carry your unlived lives. While we may give birth to our children, it is humbling to note that, often, they give birth to the potentialities of our souls.

Prescription of the Aditi Archetype

- Attending to the archetype of Aditi involves listening to the whispers of your soul that come through your dreams, fantasies, and daydreams, and through the creative process in poetry, prose, art, cinema, and other media.
- You can access the archetype of Aditi by creating a sacred space where you can tune in to the void. You can achieve this by cultivating solitude, silence, studio time, meditation, and journaling, and by attending to the present moment.
- Accessing Aditi involves a more advanced technique called active imagination, which we will discuss later in the book.
- One important method to invoke the latent code of Aditi is to honor your creative process, or the fourth quadrant of your life.

You must honor the fourth quadrant of creativity to balance the other three quadrants of love, work, and play.

- The biggest step toward activating Aditi is to evolve a reflective and symbolic attitude toward life. This involves respecting and exploring the meaning behind the outer manifestations of your life and relationships. You then become attuned to the whispers of your soul in all aspects of your life—events, relationships, problems, your creative process, and your medical and psychiatric symptoms.

- A method I have found clinically and personally useful in engaging the void and creating a Healing Zone is to imagine the void as a circular image and use that image to explore what emerges from the void. This emergent image is the *mandala* of new consciousness, the prescription and instruction from your soul to create new life consciousness out of the void. Some patients have found that creating a collage from magazine clippings is a useful exercise.

Ganesha

Another archetype guiding the transit through the Healing Zone is the elephant-headed god Ganesha, one of the most revered deities in India in his role as the remover of obstacles and guide to auspicious new beginnings (see figure 10). My personal encounter with Ganesha started in the mid-1990s, when my daughter, Ami, and I visited India. It was a very long and tiring journey. In Mumbai on the first night, we relaxed and went for a stroll. Somehow in this huge, frenetic metropolis that is unlike anywhere else on the planet, we ended up in a little curio shop. A small statue of Ganesha intrigued my daughter. It was made of solid cast silver and, at first glance, did not even look balanced enough to stay upright. It had an inexplicable charm, however, so we paid too much for it and took it home. Since that moment, the symbol of Ganesha has come alive in

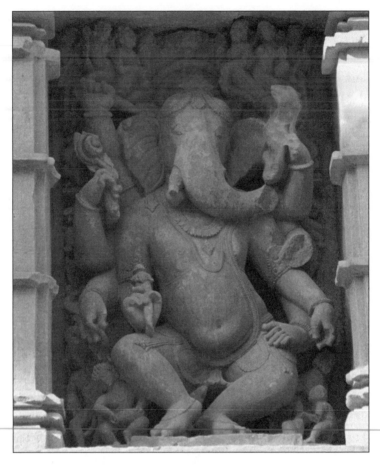

Figure 10. Ganesha, archetype of new beginnings.

my life. In order to illustrate how Ganesha altered my life, however, I must first relate the story of the elephant-headed god.

Parvati, a very powerful and beautiful woman, was married to Shiva, who led a much-fractured life, alternating between spending a thousand ascetic years alone in the mountains meditating and coming home to a domestic life with his wife. He then returned to the mountains and the cycle repeated without end. In a way, I was caught up in the Shiva archetype, trapped in my medical and psychiatric world, with precious little time for my family.

While Shiva was lost in his meditative enterprise, Parvati understandably grew bored after several thousand years of neglect. One day, as she took a bath in the holy River Ganges, her frustration led to a fruitful idea. The Ganges flows from the hair of Shiva as he sits and meditates. In a sense, Shiva is the father and Parvati the adoptive mother of the Ganges. As Parvati bathed in the river, she decided she must have a companion. So she took some of her skin rubbings and threw them into the river. Out came a very handsome young man called Ganesha in his mammoth cosmic form. To pacify those around him, however, he assumed human form.

Ganesha and his mother, Parvati, lived in a cave and had a very peaceful and playful time together. Parvati wasn't lonely anymore now that she had her son as a companion. One day, she was taking a bath and instructed her son to guard the cave so no one could enter while she was undressed. Unfortunately, Shiva chose that very day, of all the hundreds of years that he had been away, to return to the cave looking for his wife. Ganesha, who was guarding the cave, refused Shiva entry. Shiva was very angry and cut off Ganesha's head with his sword, not knowing that this was his own son. When Parvati came out and saw what had happened, she was extremely despondent and grief-stricken.

Parvati—like Demeter, the Greek mother goddess whose daughter, Persephone, was kidnapped by Hades and carried to the Underworld—went into extended mourning and the entire universe came to a standstill. The gods pleaded with Shiva to reverse his sentence and restore Ganesha's life. Eventually, Shiva made a compromise. Ganesha could not have his old head back, but the next creature that walked past Shiva would be sacrificed and its head placed on Ganesha's body.

The next creature that passed was an elephant, and Shiva kept his word. He took the elephant's head and put it on the body of his son. That is why Ganesha manifests in the form in which we now know him—with the head of an elephant. He was reborn as an auspicious god of new beginnings.

The Ganesha archetype carries three lessons. First, it teaches that the spark of possibility can grow in boredom and the void. Often, we engage the Healing Zone when we experience what the ego considers to be boredom and what the soul experiences as a creative possibility. We meet this phenomenon time and again in our own lives and in those of creative individuals. Witness the popular story of Isaac Newton, who was sitting beneath an apple tree when an apple dropped on his head, providing inspiration for his universal theory of gravitation.

Another example is the story of Archimedes' accidental discovery. The king of Syracuse had commissioned the construction of a beautiful golden crown. When the goldsmith brought him the crown, the king suspected him of stealing some of the gold and replacing it with silver. Wanting to be sure, he asked Archimedes to discover the true content of the crown. Archimedes pondered the problem for some time and, one fateful morning in the baths of Syracuse, he found the answer.

Stepping into his tub, Archimedes noticed that this action caused some of the water to spill over. He suddenly realized that the volume of the water being displaced equaled the volume of his body in the tub. He was so excited by the revelation that he ran through the streets naked, yelling: "Eureka," or "I found it!" He believed that he could measure the volume of any irregular solid by placing it in water and calculating the amount of water it displaced. He solved the king's problem by placing equal weights of gold and silver in water. The silver had a greater volume because it displaced more water. That meant that the silver was less dense than the gold, because it had the same weight but a larger volume. Archimedes then compared a lump of gold to the crown. The two had the same weight, but when Archimedes measured their volumes, the crown's was larger. Therefore, the crown was less dense and not made of pure gold. The king, now knowing that the goldsmith had replaced some of the gold in the crown with silver, had him executed.

The second lesson of the Ganesha archetype is that, when you encounter adversity—an accident, a major loss, a beheading of the old system—it may feel like the end of your world. However, if you remember that Ganesha is at work, it opens up interesting possibilities of new creation via the Healing Zone. During the recession of 2008, I was heartened to learn that many of my patients and friends had to let go of comfortable but soulless jobs, but that they were able to use this crisis to engage professions they had really wanted all their lives.

The third lesson of Ganesha is that we must always be ready for a new head, a new attitude, a new way of thinking and being.

So how did I find Ganesha? After my daughter and I returned from India, my wife vocalized her dream of many years to open a restaurant. With the help of my daughter, this wish became reality. The two of them painstakingly reviewed a list of names for the restaurant, much as people do when naming a child. They chose to call it Dancing Ganesha. The name was fitting, but, at that time, I hadn't yet made the connection with the myth and the symbol of Ganesha.

Soon this mother-daughter enterprise became a flourishing reality. Remember, Ganesha was formed in a collaboration between mother and daughter—Parvati and the Ganges. That mythic symbol was lived out in my own life as a collaboration between mother and daughter as well, but without the father's input—my input. Like Shiva, I felt excluded from the cave. I was incensed and wanted to cut off the head of the project. What about me? They told me I had my patients and clinic, and that I could go back to my mountain.

I wasn't easily deterred, however, and did my best to sabotage the project—if only unconsciously. My wife and I finally negotiated a workable compromise in which her mission and my need for respect were both honored. Afterward, I gave full support to their business. We played out the myth of Ganesha in our own lives. The restaurant was emotionally beheaded by the male Shiva energy; then an eventual rapprochement between the masculine and the feminine made room for union and the emergence of the divine child. When masculine and feminine collaborate, the results are wondrous.

A few months later, I received a deeper indication of what motivated the beliefs my wife and daughter infused into Dancing Ganesha. When the restaurant opened, it received accolades from critics and diners. The reviews said that the food was excellent and the atmosphere beautiful, but that there was something more, something different, something unique about the place. One evening, I dined with my wife at someone else's restaurant and had an enlightening experience that gave me an insight into why she and my daughter had to start Ganesha. The restaurant we went to that night was classy, expensive, and traditional. The patrons were mostly men in suits. There were only two women in the room, quietly listening to the jokes of their loud and garrulous husbands. I wondered where the other women were. Surely, all these other men were not bachelors. Another interesting observation was that my wife and I were the only non-white people in the room. Where was the rest of America? We paid our bill and left with a strange feeling in our hearts.

It wasn't like that in my wife and daughter's restaurant. There, the patrons included single and married individuals, men and women, couples and families, white, black, and brown people, young and old, gay and straight—all together forming a rich tapestry of cultures and traditions. I had come to America in search of the great new frontier, with promises of racial equality, cultural diversity, respect for varying perspectives—a mosaic of the human race, a fractal of the promise of civilization. It was a paradox that, of all the places in America, I found it in my wife and daughter's restaurant! Such is the power of the feminine; such is the blessing of Parvati and the wonders of her creative divine child, Ganesha.

Prescriptions of the Ganesha Archetype

- Losing your head, as in the Ganesha myth, is the sacrifice you must make to move from illness to wellness. On your path to the soul, guided by Parvati and the archetype of the goddess Shakti, you must be prepared to make the necessary sacrifice to find your higher nature. This involves letting go of old habits and business as usual.

- What does it mean to have the head of an elephant? What does that experience feel like? An elephant's head is close to the heavens; its trunk is close to the earth. This symbolizes the union of these two extremes—the cosmic and the human. When you bridge your shadow with the light in your nature—your spiritual potential with your frail human existence, your outer with your inner life, action with reflection—your darkest and highest potential unite and you live out your Ganesha potential.

- The myth of Ganesha is one framework through which you can negotiate the boundaries between masculine and feminine in the culture and in your psyche. This myth is a gift of Parvati. Even though Shiva promised the gods not to procreate in order to maintain political balance, Parvati managed to activate Shiva's procreative potential through Ganesha. Similarly in contemporary culture, when men sacrifice their creative potential for political and survival expediency, the power of the goddess Parvati helps the masculine realize its true potential.

- Ganesha advises you to make compromises. It was not possible for Shiva to undo his decision to decapitate his son, but the couple was able to negotiate a compromise—an elephant head instead.

- The guidance of Ganesha and the various steps in this archetype are valuable prescriptions for harvesting the full potential of the Healing Zone, where you embark on new beginnings. For example, you must examine each issue, not only with your elephant head up in the sky—your intuitive function—but also with your trunk close to the ground—your sensate function or attention to small details.

Hermes

Hermes, or Mercury, is the messenger god, the divine herald from the unconscious who mediates the crossroad between consciousness and the unconscious—

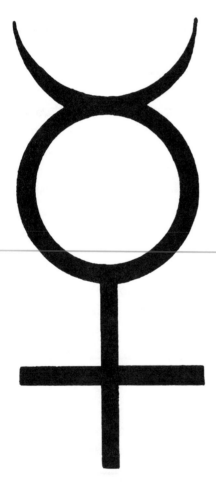

between transitional states of consciousness (see figure 11). This fleet-footed messenger transmits the healing wisdom of the universe to our human psyches by connecting two or more states of consciousness. He mediates between wakefulness and sleep, and between sleep and dreams, bringing wakefulness and dreams together in meditative states of consciousness. He also mediates between the mind and the body.

Hermes is the analogue of Asclepius, the patron god of physicians who presides over the Healing Zone. The familiar symbol of medicine, the caduceus, originated in the worship of Hermes/Asclepius and symbolizes the union of two states of consciousness to form a third state, the Healing Zone (see figure 12).

Figure 11. Hermes, patron god of the Healing Zone.

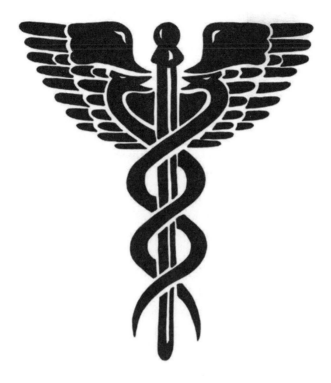

Figure 12. The caduceus, familiar symbol of medicine.

Hermes is the god of shepherds, land travel, merchants, weights and measures, oratory, literature, athletics, and thieves. He is a patron of poets and is known for his cunning and shrewdness. Most important, he is the messenger of the gods.

According to legend, Hermes was born in a cave on Mount Cyllene in Arcadia. Zeus had impregnated Maia in the dead of night while all the other gods slept. Hermes, the child of this union, was born miraculously as dawn broke. Maia wrapped him in swaddling clothes and fell fast asleep. Hermes, however, squirmed free and ran off to Thessaly, where Apollo, his brother, grazed his cattle. Hermes stole a number of the herd and drove them back to Greece. He hid them in a small grotto near the city of Pylos and covered their tracks. Before returning to the cave, Hermes caught a tortoise, killed it, and removed its entrails. Using the intestines from a cow stolen from Apollo and the hollow tortoise shell, he made the first lyre. When he reached the cave, he wrapped himself back up in the swaddling bands.

When Apollo realized he had been robbed, he protested to Maia that Hermes had taken his cattle. Maia looked at Hermes and said that could not be, as he was still wrapped in his swaddling clothes. Zeus the All-Powerful intervened, saying that he had been watching, that Hermes had in fact stolen the cattle, and that he should return them to Apollo. As the argument went on, Hermes began to play his lyre. The sweet music enchanted Apollo and he offered Hermes the cattle in exchange for the lyre, which became one of Apollo's symbols. Later, while Hermes watched over his herd, he invented the pipes known as the syrinx (pan pipes), which are made from reeds. (He is also credited with inventing the flute, which Apollo also coveted.) So Hermes bartered with Apollo, who gave his golden wand in return for the pipes. Hermes later used this wand as his herald's staff.

As messenger of the gods, it was Hermes' duty to guide the souls of the dead to the Underworld. He was also closely associated with bringing dreams to mortals. Hermes is usually depicted with a broad-brimmed hat or a winged cap and winged sandals, clutching his staff (*kerykeion* in Greek, *caduceus* in Latin). His clothes were usually those of a traveler or those of a workman or shepherd.

Prescriptions of the Hermes Archetype

- The Hermes archetype is crucial for understanding the workings of the Healing Zone. To engage the dynamics of growth and healing, you must learn to make compromises between the different parts of your mind and different sectors of your life, just as Hermes compromised with Apollo by making a deal—a lyre for the cattle; the pipes for the wand. This creates a win-win dynamic.

- My patients often complain that, in their busy lives, they do not have time for mindfulness, meditation, yoga, reflection, and inner life. This is usually an accurate reflection of their outer reality. On closer examination, however, I have found that part of the problem is the difficulty they have setting priorities. The Hermes archetype helps you set priorities between the competing aspects of your life.

- In my personal and clinical experience, perfectionism is a strong pretext for procrastination. Perfectionists often hide behind the axiom that, if they can't do something perfectly, they would rather not do it at all. These individuals create such an impossible threshold of assessment for themselves, others, and the world that it becomes a pretext for inactivity, passivity, procrastination, and complacency. Hermes is an imperfect god, a thief who stole Apollo's golden cattle. However, his imperfection opened a dialogue between the Hermetic and the Apollonian aspects of the psyche—that is, a compromise between action and perfection. Imperfect action is symbolized by Hermes; perfection is symbolized by Apollo.

- An intervention I have found helpful for obsessive perfectionists is the 80/20 rule. The value of the 80/20 rule is that it reminds you to focus on the 20 percent that matters, rather than the 80 percent that doesn't. Of the things you do during your day, only 20 percent really matter. That 20 percent produces 80 percent of your results. Identify and focus on those things. This implies working smart, not just working hard. When you work smart, you eliminate redundancy in your life and focus on what really matters. This makes room for self-care and engaging the Healing Zone. Hermes helps you focus on the 20 percent that counts, while letting go of the 80 percent that is redundant or irrelevant. Authentic compromise is only possible when both parties focus on the 20 percent that matters.

- By negotiating between different realms, Hermes represents building bridges between different sectors of your life. This means balancing love, work, play, creativity, and spirituality. We often lead lopsided lives without adequate representations of all the sectors that need a vote in our lives to establish a democracy of health and wholeness.

- In challenging your perfectionism, Hermes guides you to entertain the give-and-take in life. You can't do everything to perfection. Compromises must be made. You may not be capable of being a perfect professional and a perfect parent. Your enterprise must be good enough, but not perfect. If you can't do meditation every day, settle for every three days. If you can't execute a perfect project at work, settle for a functionally viable project, provided that yours or someone else's life does not depend upon it. In observing mentors that I admire, I have noticed that they give it all they have in trying to help their students and their patients in their academic and clinical work, but often their clinical notes are less than perfect. Their priority is helping others, not writing perfect soulless charts. Hermes is an imperfect god, a thief, and a trickster. But he is a great negotiator who gets the job done.

- The final prescription of the Hermes archetype is the pyramid of your personal priorities. God is first; you are second; all others are third. By placing yourself second, below only God, you are able to attend to yourself properly. When you are in optimal health, you are more available to others whom you are privileged to serve and love. Hermes guides you to establish this pyramid in negotiating your priorities.

- In summary, Hermes guides you to maintain a life/work balance and give adequate representation on the stage of consciousness to all five sectors of your life: love, work, play, creativity, and spirituality.

Bardo: Death and Healing

In Tibetan, *bar* means "between"; *do* means "two." *Bardo* thus alludes to the state between death and rebirth, the transitional or intermediate state of consciousness akin to the Hindu concept of the gap, or *Turiya*—the Healing Zone. Just as Ganesha is the archetype of new beginnings, the *Tibetan Book of the Dead,* or *Bardo Thodol* (Jung, 1960), offers us a template of the archetype of death and its potential to set us free from the suffering of the human condition. It is meant to be a guide for those who have died as they transition from their former lives to a new destination (see figure 13).

Death is an archetypal event. It is a constant of life. Everything born must die at some point. According to the Hindu scriptures, even our universe endures death and rebirth every 400 billion years and each of us undergoes the cycle of birth, death, and reincarnation. Hindus believe that, in each lifetime, we create positive or negative karma based on the choices we make. When we live according to our spiritual purpose, or dharma, we create positive karma. This is how a young soul matures and becomes an old soul worthy of merger with Spirit or the divine, finally breaking the repetitive cycle of reincarnation and attaining moksha, or freedom from the human condition, thus merging with the divine flow.

The Buddhist tradition deals with the archetype of death or endings in a soulful manner. It teaches us the art of dying. The experience of death offers us a window into the realm of Spirit. If we use this window to step into the flow of the universe, we may step out of the repetitive cycle of death and rebirth and align ourselves with the flow of Spirit. *The Tibetan Book of the Dead* explores the archetype of death in three stages: *Chikka Bardo*, *Chonyid Bardo*, and *Sidpa Bardo*. Each contains its own prescriptions for wellness. Exploring the symbolic instructions of this ancient text helps us deal, not just with literal death, but also with death-like experiences—endings, losses, and disappointments—in ways that open the path from illness to wellness.

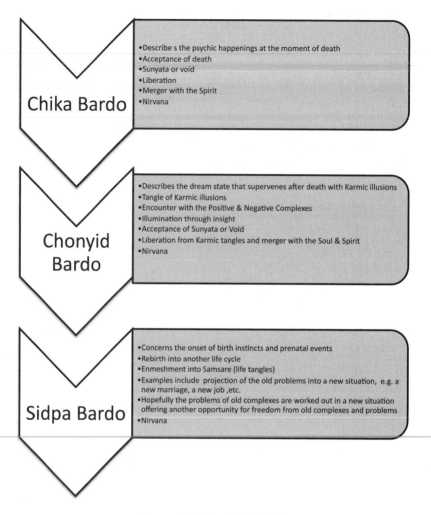

Figure 13. Bardo Thadol.

Chikka Bardo involves psychic happenings at the moment of death. Supreme insight and illumination, and hence the potential of attaining liberation, are possible during the process of dying. In Chikka Bardo, the soul (Atman) can be restored to the continuity it lost with Spirit (Brahmana) at the moment of birth.

If the Atman is not yet an old soul worthy of merger with the divine, it must go through Chonyid Bardo. In psychoanalytical terms, this means working through the complexes that get in the way. If you are unable to work through your complexes, the only venue available to you is rebirth into another life cycle, giving you another opportunity to mature into an old soul.

This happens in the third stage, Sidpa Bardo, which refers to a new beginning—analogous to a second marriage or a new career—for working out your unresolved karmic tangles. However, for many people this means merely changing the actors, not rewriting the play. The outcome of the "new experience" will be identical to your previous experience unless you work through your dysfunctions. Unless you change your own attitude, the outcome will be the same.

Chonyid Bardo is an after-death dream state suffused with karmic illusions. Our unresolved complexes get hold of the psyche and the possibility of Nirvana wanes as we move farther from the illumination of Chikka Bardo and inch toward reincarnation or rebirth. In Chonyid Bardo, the dead person encounters the wrathful and peaceful deities representing the positive and negative complexes that Buddhist thought subsumes under the concept of *samsara,* or entanglement in the *maya* of existence—as opposed to entering *sunyata,* or the void where the soul's slate is wiped clean and readied for merger with Spirit.

The third state, Sidpa Bardo, concerns the onset of birth instincts and prenatal events. Freudian analysis explores Sidpa Bardo through the lens of parental relations and sexual fantasies. Jung believed that, if Freud had delved deeper into the prenatal psyche and intrauterine experiences, he might have uncovered the existence of the soul and the process of rebirth as a way to work through residual complexes, enabling the ego to mature into a deeper state of consciousness. Clinically, this is akin to helping individuals who have been unable or unwilling to learn from their life experiences, and have repeated their cycle of mistakes in every new job or relationship, only to realize, finally, that the problem lies in their own attitudes, character defects, and maladaptive life patterns.

Prescriptions of the Bardo Archetype

- Life-changing events—the death of a loved one, a health crisis, the end of a significant relationship, the loss of a job—all offer death-like experiences. You may be tempted to recreate what you have lost with a new job or relationship, but unless you take time to step out of this repetitive cycle and reflect with the goal of resetting your life and attitude—in other words, embrace the Chikka state—you will recreate the same dysfunction in a different garb.

- A reflective exploration of the contribution you make to your own problems can be undertaken in therapy or self-reflection; it is guided by the Chonyid stage of Bardo. Here, you encounter your own inner demons and angels and modulate them so that they are worthy of assimilation into your personality as part of the solution rather than the problem.

- If you can't entirely let go of the old attitudes that cause you difficulty, as in Chikka Bardo, or can't understand your own contribution to your problems in Chonyid Bardo, your only choice is the Sidpa state of rebirth into another job, marriage, or health problem—which gives you yet another learning cycle. The pattern will continue until you get it right!

In the next chapter, we will explore the interplay of archetypes and consciousness with the structure of the brain and the nervous system.

Chapter 3

Engaging the Healing Zone

The starting point in the journey into the Healing Zone is your personal goal for wellness. Are you seeking to heal a particular illness, ailment, complex, or relationship? Or are you seeking a higher degree of spiritual awareness? Once you have identified your goal, write it down in your journal before you immerse yourself in the depths of the Healing Zone.

Next, identify your physical, emotional, relational, or spiritual focus for intervention. If you hope to attend to a medical problem like chronic back pain, you must focus on the physical body. If you are concerned with an emotional problem like panic attacks, you must focus on the mind. If your concerns are related to intellectual or cognitive distortions like catastrophizing or personalizing, you must focus on cognitive restructuring. If your focus is on moving from a horizontal to a vertical axis of existence, from an ego-driven life to a soul-driven life, your focus must be to cultivate a spiritual attitude.

Once you have established a focus for intervention based on your starting point, you must engage with the fourth state of consciousness, the Healing Zone.

For most individuals, the Healing Zone operates unconsciously; sometimes, however, an actual symbol will appear, offering to solve the riddle of your illness. Jennifer, a patient with a thyroid disorder, discovered an image of her father choking her whenever she tried to speak of her childhood. While her father never actually tried to choke her, he was a bully and a domineering tyrant who could not tolerate his children speaking unless spoken to. As a result, Jennifer was stuck in her fifth, or throat, chakra, unable to express her authentic voice. This insight and image helped her gradually reclaim her authentic voice and self-assertiveness.

Once your connection with the Healing Zone has been established, it is crucial to keep up the practice of regular engagement with this aspect of your consciousness. With regular practice, you can maintain a sacred alchemical healing vessel that pours out the ambrosia of life and vitality. This becomes the Holy Grail that nourishes and enriches you, and connects you with the grace of the healing flow of the universe.

Julie is a middle-aged professional with symptoms of depression and chronic low-back pain. Her orthopedic consultant recommended back surgery. She decided to wait until she better understood the dynamic of the symptoms. We applied the methods of transcendental meditation to her back pain. Her image of that malady involved carrying a large sack on her back. When we entered the Healing Zone, the image of the sack was amplified into the archetypal image of Atlas, the mythical hero who carries the weight of the world on his back. The new image she discovered in the Healing Zone helped her understand the origins of her condition; she was then able to free herself from a sense of responsibility as the caretaker of everyone around her. The Atlas insight allowed her to let go of her caretaker complex. Julie is much improved and surgery has not been necessary.

Robert was struggling with grief and depression. He dreamed that he held his dog, Rusty, in his arms. We decided to honor the dream by immersing it in the Healing Zone, holding the dream image of Rusty together with a conscious image of the dog in the therapy session. We then decided to deepen the image into Robert's emotional body. At once, Robert remembered that his dream recalled that Rusty had died in his arms after a bout with cancer—a painful experience for Robert. We stayed with the image in his consciousness as he re-experienced the loss and the grief it recalled. Then we invited Rusty to guide us as to why he had incarnated in Robert's dream.

Soon, Robert had an insight. In a few weeks, his son and his family, who had stayed with Robert for a year while between jobs, were moving out of his house to their new home. Robert was very attached to his grandchild and the impending move recalled the loss of Rusty. The dream image of Rusty was both a reminder of that loss and a reassurance that Rusty's memory was with him during this transition. This consciousness of loss and grief led to an awareness of the freedom that comes with the empty-nest syndrome. Once Robert became conscious of his grief about the empty nest, his depression abated; he was able to grieve, but was free to pursue other creative goals while maintaining a robust connection with his grandchildren.

The Triune Brain

In his groundbreaking research, Dr. Paul MacLean laid out our contemporary understanding of the human brain and its structure, function, and origins (MacLean, 1990). Through a comparative study of existing vertebrates and fossil records, he outlined how the present human brain evolved from our early ancestors, including reptiles and lower mammals. The three "layers" of the brain—the reptilian brain, the paleomammalian or limbic brain, and the neomammalian brain or neocortical nervous system—have their own autonomy and functions and lead to highly complex and adaptive responses to our environment.

The oldest layer, the reptilian brain, orchestrates our basic survival needs. The limbic brain houses archetypal memory and emotions and is where mammals evolved their maternal and attachment functions for nurturing their loved ones. The neocortical brain adds the functions of discernment and will. It is responsible for cognitive function, intellectual capacity, speech, and voluntary motor function (see figure 14).

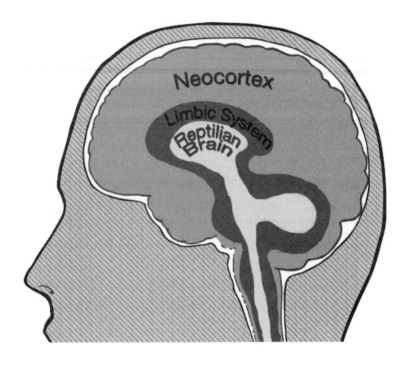

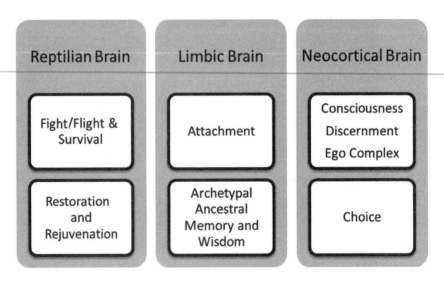

Figure 14. The triune brain.

Most of modern psychiatry tends to focus on the neocortical layer, or our cognitive functions. The Jungian approach goes deeper into the limbic, archetypal context of our experience. Ancient Hindu healing traditions focus on these two layers, but tend to go to the roots of the reptilian layer to effect healing and wholeness. The ancient traditions of Ayurvedic medicine—pranayama, yoga, and transcendental meditation—help to reset the reptilian nervous system for the deepest healing of the mind and the body. The Healing Zone is meant to bridge all three brain layers and hold them in consciousness to help with healing. For example, in pranayama, we engage the reptilian brain through regulating breathing while simultaneously holding a healing image that activates the limbic archetypal consciousness.

In Western medicine, the emphasis is on neocortical healing, in that all treatments must conform to intellectual, evidence-based systems of care. It thus treats groups rather than unique individuals. Its standardized protocols work well for setting theoretical norms, but not as well for establishing the narrative of a unique life. While the Western medical tradition has made substantial contributions to treating the symptoms of illness, it often neglects its underlying cause. Thus the illness returns, creating a cycle of illness, medication, procedures, side effects, and more intervention—an endless loop of illness and intervention in a medical-industrial matrix. So how can healers break this vicious cycle? Here, the ancient healing traditions have much to offer in moving us from illness to wellness.

Attending to Your Three Brains

- Experts have outlined several measures to monitor a person's reptilian brain, which regulates the autonomic health status, including measuring the resting heart rate, heart-rate variability, heart-rate recovery after exercise, and heart-rate turbulence. While some of these methods require laboratory settings, you can easily monitor your resting pulse rate and your rate of recovery after exercise or exertion. A resting rate in the 60s to 70s indicates good autonomic health, while a rate in the 80s or 90s signals trouble. The longer the peak rate takes to return to the resting pulse rate, the more brittle your autonomic nervous system.

> *Never forget the importance of the pulse! Before practicing any of the suggestions and exercises offered in this book, record your resting pulse rate and peak pulse-rate recovery time after strenuous physical or mental activity.*

- The health of your limbic brain manifests in your attention to your personal myth or the archetype that guides your life journey. In the section on archetypes, I outline some of the myths that guide you in the Healing Zone. Choose the myth that best guides your personal journey at the present time. For some, it may be necessary to honor the void of the goddess Aditi; for others, it may be Bardo—the death of a certain dysfunctional aspect of their lives. Many may find the guidance of Ganesha helpful in making auspicious new beginnings. Some may find the archetype of the transitional zone—the Lion Man—helpful and use the practice that engages this zone—meditation. When caught in the tight spots, crossroads, or dilemmas of life, the guidance of the divine Trickster, Hermes, is invaluable.
- The health of the neocortical brain is assessed by challenging your cognitive distortions, replacing them with rational thoughts, and invoking the ego functions of suppression, altruism, anticipation, sublimation, humor, reflective function, and symbolic attitude.

The Spiritual Attitude

One of the prerequisites of engaging the Healing Zone is the spiritual attitude that lies at the core of all ancient healing traditions. A spiritual or symbolic attitude toward life that moves you from the horizontal to the vertical axis of consciousness is essential to wellness. You must balance the mundane with the sacred dimension of your life and acknowledge Spirit as the source of your wellness. A spiritual attitude invites the wisdom of the universe into your healing practice and invokes the guidance of the archetypes. Without it, the Healing Zone becomes just a mumbo-jumbo exercise or a parlor game.

Characteristics of the spiritual attitude include:

- Belief that a deeper center of consciousness, the soul, guides your inner life and the bigger picture of your life, while your ego manages your dealings with daily responsibilities and the outer life.
- Belief that the soul (Atman) is connected to the universal consciousness of Spirit (Brahmana).
- Awareness of the eternal dance between soul and Spirit. The soul gets its instructions from Spirit in guiding your life.
- Openness to the whispers of your soul in guiding your life onto its spiritual path.
- Respect for dreams, daydreams, fantasies, art and creativity, physical and mental symptoms, accidents, chance events, hang-ups, and relationship problems as the whispers of your soul.
- A reflective attitude and the ability to understand problems as passwords connecting your outer life with your soul, and your soul with Spirit.
- Respect for the unknown. Your soul lives at the boundary between what you know consciously and the unknown precinct where Spirit begins.

- The capacity to deal with uncertainty so you are able to understand the symbolic meaning of how a situation connects you with your soul and, through your soul, with Spirit.
- Respect for the symbols that emerge from your unconscious to inform your life and align it with Spirit's calling.
- Establishment of a personal framework to maintain a dialogue with soul and Spirit. This includes a personal system to decode, honor, and implement the intent of the symbols that emerge from your soul to guide your life.
- A framework of mindfulness practice that helps you stay present in the moment without getting stuck in experiences from the past or expectations of the future.
- A reflective attitude that opens you up to investigate the true nature of every moment and its meaning in the flow of the universe. This quiets the mind and leads to purpose, focus, tranquility, and an experience of wellness.

Over many ages, the collective wisdom of humanity has accumulated in our myths. These myths play out in our individual lives as life patterns, dreams, and medical and psychiatric symptoms, as well as in our art and creative products. Spirit also modulates this accumulated human wisdom. Whenever you are dealing with major issues—initiations, developments, crises, transitions, or catastrophes—this collective wisdom can be activated to guide you. The spiritual attitude is respectful of these guiding and healing archetypes and open to their input in our lives.

The first step in receiving the gifts of healing and recovery from Spirit is to empty the cup of your consciousness and ego, making room for your soul. An empty cup makes room for the recreation of consciousness with new images, energies, and potentials. A cluttered life and a muddled mind block the emergence of new and adaptive psychic structures.

Emptying the full cup of your life involves letting go of your complexes, hang-ups, and character defects—including perfectionism, narcissism, histrionics, avoidance, self-defeating behaviors, paranoia, withdrawal, intrusiveness, dependency, medical and psychiatric symptoms, obsessions, compulsions, and addictive behaviors. These may involve alcohol, drugs, food, sex, gambling, pornography, holding grudges and resentments, grief over old losses, envy, dysfunctional attitudes and beliefs, hurtful attachments, enmeshed and dysfunctional relationships, codependency on another for self-esteem, and life goals that have outlived their purpose. You cannot begin to empty your cup until you recognize and let go of these elements in your life. Most important, emptying your cup involves letting go of the past, engaging the present, and making room for the future.

While it may not be possible to empty your cup at the first few attempts, the movement from illness to wellness begins with being conscious of this task and undertaking it with baby steps, in small increments, one day at a time. Gradually, you will gain ground in this apparently uneven battle. This is a courageous journey of recovery that calls for patience, perseverance, and persistence against the power of the dark side of your own nature. If you persist in this hero's journey, the healing forces of the universe will step in to guide your path toward health and wellness.

The psychological term for this phenomenon is *kenosis*. Kenosis is the concept of self-emptying and becoming entirely receptive to God and his perfect will. The Buddhist tradition talks of the need to empty the cup of life to receive the gifts of the universe. In Christianity, kenosis denotes the relinquishment of the form of God by Jesus in becoming man. When you relinquish your old dysfunctional ways of doing and being, you make room for the grace of divine consciousness to incarnate in your life.

To move from illness to wellness, you must live in the present, notice the whispers of your soul, and make time to reflect. The human mind chatters. There's always something going on in your mind. It's like a busy street corner in a metropolis, with emotions, thoughts, hopes, fears, and memories crisscrossing and colliding with each other, tugging at your attention and distracting you from your focus. To be in the present, you have to do two things simultaneously: pay some attention to the chatter and maintain some degree of detachment. Your routine ego consciousness is in the experiencing-and-managing mode. The task of attending to wellness calls for the cultivation of an observing ego—a detached consciousness that can become the reflective witness to its own experience. This moves the compass of the ego from action to reflection.

Of course, you have to pay some attention to the chatter, because it is a signal from your soul. The memories, fears, hopes, regrets, and fantasies that scurry through your thoughts are not without importance. The emotional coloration and intensity of your thoughts signifies the specific content of your consciousness.

A degree of distance—the "observing ego"—is vital, however. Total disconnection from emotion leaves only your rational mind on the job. Feeling is a function of the incarnated individual soul, and you need to be aware of your feelings if you are to attend to your soul. Only when you are able to observe and to feel simultaneously do you have the possibility of understanding the messages of the soul. If you let the heavy traffic that sometimes fills your mind run you down or carry you away, you lose the necessary degree of detachment.

The second necessary element for moving from illness to wellness is noticing the whispers of your soul. You must take time to reflect actively on what is going on in your life—both your outer and inner lives. You must also make space in your busy life for active reflection. It's as important as regularly brushing your teeth. Active reflection is a habit you need to form. It means that you must stop, look, and listen *before* the alarm goes off—*before* a complex erupts, *before* a relationship goes sour, *before* you fall ill.

The third prerequisite for attending to your soul is time. You must take time to notice what is going on and reflect on what you notice. When an emotionally colored thought, image, or experience of whatever degree of intensity completely fills your consciousness, you do not have the degree of detachment necessary to reflect on it. Setting aside time for reflection, safe from intrusion and distraction, creates the sacred space in which you can ponder the whispers of your soul and explore their meaning for your life.

Establishing and maintaining this three-part foundation—being in the present, noticing the whispers of the soul, and making time to reflect—presents an ongoing challenge. You won't get it perfect the first time. All three elements demand your patience and discipline. With practice, however, you can steadily improve your skills and increase your harvest of insight. Use the spiritual quotient assessment below to help you on this path.

Spiritual Quotient Assessment

1. Do you feel that you live your life primarily as a conscious enterprise, or do you have a sense of some deeper source, some unconscious dimension that has some impact on your life and its direction?

2. Do you have any method or system through which to make a connection with your inner life?

3. Are you able to use your dreams as a method to maintain dialogue with your inner life?

4. Are you able to perceive obstacles and disappointments in your life, not only as setbacks, but potentially also as whispers of your inner life trying to point you in directions you may not have consciously considered?

5. When you are confronted with medical or psychiatric problems, relationship difficulties, your own hang-ups or shortcomings, family problems, failures, or adversity, do you see these as difficulties to be overcome as soon as possible? Or do you feel that these hold important clues from which you can learn to live a more spiritually informed and meaningful life?

6. As you review your life journey so far, do you feel that all your successes, failures, and detours have revolved around some central theme, as if some invisible force or trajectory were guiding you?

7. Do you have some dawning awareness of a deeper sense of purpose in your life guided by some inner wisdom?

8. As you look back on your life so far, do you have an awareness that, as you were busy pursuing your goals, some unintended life pattern has been emerging? Does this unplanned life pattern have some central theme, meaning, or purpose? How is this pattern at variance with your consciously established life goals?

9. How much of your life is based on the demands of outer realities? How much do you reflect on some aspect of your deeper, inner, unconscious life and factor it into your deliberations?

10. When dealing with difficult people, problems, or decisions, do you react to the situation immediately or reflect on it and its meaning in terms of your outer and inner life before acting?

11. Do you make active efforts to reflect daily or regularly on the connection between your outer life and your inner life? How do your two worlds interface and impact each other?

12. Looking back on your life, what small and seemingly insignificant event or encounter had a significant impact on its course and direction?

13. Do you tend to focus on past problems, past glory, future problems, and possibilities? Or do you live your life in the present moment?

14. As you assess your life to date, what contribution do you feel you may have made to the community and humanity? Do you feel that, in some way, you have made this world a better place in which to live?

The Interpretation of Dreams

If mythology is the dream of a culture, individual dreams represent your personal myths and are guideposts on the path to your soul and your destiny. Usually, a dream supplies information that your consciousness either does not have, or does not adequately perceive or value. The following general overview will help you orient yourself to the interpretation of your dreams.

Dreams are an integral part of the brain function of every human being. Each night, we sleep from seven to nine hours and our sleep is divided into deep sleep, when our brain waves fluctuate between the theta state (4–8 Hz per second) and the deep sleep of delta waves (1–4 Hz per second). When in very deep sleep, we experience a burst of brain activity in the form of beta waves (12–24 Hz per second). At this stage, the body is paralyzed, but the brain is awake to its deepest, or soul, consciousness. This is called the dream stage of sleep. Rapid eye movement (REM) occurs during this stage, as if we were observing our inner world from our deepest sleep.

The dream state of sleep gives you a soul's-eye view of others, the world, the future, and yourself. It is as if you took a troubling or perplexing aspect of your present life situation and Googled it using the cosmic Internet. Dreams factor in all the wisdom, archetypal guidance, and ancestral data that your psyche can bring to bear on the questions you are dealing with in your outer life. Dreams are a crucial and precious consultation from the soul and the universe on the perplexing dilemmas of your life. You ignore the guidance of dreams at your own peril (Johnson, 1989).

Dreams by themselves are not within the Healing Zone of consciousness. However, when considered consciously and respectfully, they yield guidance and create a new consciousness on your path to wellness. Remembering a dream is only the first step into this new state, however. Holding the content of the dream in specific ways in your consciousness, under the gaze of your observing ego, is the crucial next step toward new insights. You can't just simply cut, mix, and heat ingredients to make a gourmet meal; they must be prepared in a specific way to create a culinary masterpiece.

Dream interpretation dates back to ancient times and can be found in the sacred literature of many cultures. The Second Book of Daniel includes a detailed account of how the prophet interpreted King Nebuchadnezzar's dreams. The ancient Greeks acknowledged the value of dreams in the Asclepian healing tradition. When a physician was unable to cure an illness, he turned for help to the god of healing, Asclepius. The Greeks believed that answers came through a visitation in dreams from the healing god (or one of his totems, a dog or snake). The dream resulted either in a spontaneous healing or an indication of what had to be done to effect a cure. In temples to the god, *therapeutes* (therapists) conveyed the sick to chambers where they prayed and fell into sleep, expecting a dream visitation from Asclepius. Illnesses cured in this way were recorded on thousands of votive offerings presented to the temples.

Aristotle was one of the first writers to attempt a systematic study of the mind in all its aspects, including the subtleties of sleep and dreams. Aristotle defined imagination as the result of sensory and subjective perception occurring after the disappearance of the sensed object in the form of powerful and realistic after-images. He carried this insight into the realm of sleep and applied it to dreaming. He added that, while awake, we easily distinguish between external and imagined objects. In sleep, however, this faculty disappears or is almost completely absent. As a result, we have a sense of enormous reality in dreams and the feeling that we are seeing actual events and people. Freud called this the hallucinatory property of dreams.

Dream sleep emerged 130 million years ago as a neuropsychic activity of great biological significance. EEG records in sleeping cats and humans reveal that REM sleep originates in the limbic and reptilian centers of the brain. Researchers in the 1970s (Hall, 1972) collected 50,000 dreams and identified common themes among them, including pursuit by predatory animals and hostile strangers, flying, falling, strangers, landscapes, sex, getting married, having children, taking an examination, undergoing an ordeal, traveling, swimming, watching fires, and confinement underground. These typical dreams express the shared concerns, preoccupations, and interests of all dreamers. They constitute the universal constants of the human psyche and reflect our adaptation to our primeval, hunter-gatherer roots.

According to Freud, dreams represent the gratification of an unfulfilled, infantile wish. Freud's theory of dream interpretation emphasizes the concepts of dramatization, condensation, displacement, secondary elaboration, and dream symbols that disguise the latent content of a repressed wish, making it acceptable to the consciousness without being censored by the observing, critical, moral superego.

Jung, however, defined dreams as the soul's depiction in symbolic form of the contents of the unconscious. Dreams thus have a causal and purposeful perspective. They are trying to tell us something and to guide us somewhere. Jung saw dreams as commentaries on our personal complexes. To him, our complexes and not our dreams are the royal road to the unconscious; and our complexes are the architects of dreams and symptoms. Dreams speak both to the complexes and to our unconscious commentary on the complexes. Along with the technique of free association in interpreting dreams, Jung stressed the importance of myth, history, and other cultural material as the fabric from which dreams are spun.

Jung distinguished between the subjective level, where dream figures are personifications of components of the dreamer's own psyche, and the objective level, which is inhabited by human figures that may be known to the dreamer. He believed that dreams have a prospective aspect; they can be an unconscious anticipation of a future achievement, but in the form of a preliminary sketch rather than a prophecy. Dreams are an expression of facts that are still unconscious. Unlike Freud, Jung believed that dreams do not disguise, but rather express, the unconscious in their own symbolic language.

Jung proposed four stages in the narrative of dreams;

- Exposition—the setting, place, and protagonists, and the initial situation
- Development—action, plot complications, and development of tension
- Climax—the culmination where a change in situation occurs
- Lysis—the solution or outcome signifying the prescription of the soul

Jung emphasized the context for the dream, the situation in which the dream's images are embedded, including personal associations and archetypal parallels, the immediate and the long-term conscious situation of the dreamer, and whether the dream is ongoing or part of a series.

You must make no assumptions, however, about the meaning of a dream or any of its specific images. A dream is not a psychic ruse, but a psychic fact. The personality of the dreamer and the interpreter must be considered. A dream probably does not tell you what to do; it only provides expert consultation. It must be characterized as subjective or objective. Jung recommends that you identify the problem or complex with which the dream is concerned, ascertain your relevant conscious situation, and consider whether the dream is prospective, traumatic, telepathic, or prophetic.

A Jungian dream interpretation is a hypothesis based on translating the dream as it relates to your conscious situation. The interpretation is repeatedly tested against the dream and your own situation, modified when necessary, and verified with reference to your immediate and delayed response to the dream and its interpretation. Jung's technique focuses less on free association than on a conscious illumination of chains of association directly connected with the dream images. For him, the dream is not a façade; rather, the manifest picture contains the latent meaning.

I cannot stress enough that every Jungian dream interpretation is hypothetical. An interpretation can be substantiated by a series of dreams and subsequent dreams may correct the potential mistakes made in interpretation. Jung encouraged dream journaling, including a record of successive interpretations. Gradually, you must learn self-interpretation as a way to consult your own unconscious.

Dreams give information about the secrets of your inner life and personality, in terms of both problems and potentials. Unattended, the information they give can manifest as psychological or physical symptoms. Dream analysis permits mutual assimilation of unconscious and conscious aspects of the psyche. Neither your consciousness nor the unconscious is in charge; they must collaborate. Interpretations seldom result in "this-or-that" answers; rather they yield "this-*and*-that" responses. They require exact knowledge of your situation, and the status quo of your consciousness. Dream symbolism also demands the context of your philosophical, religious, and moral convictions. Dream symbols are not disguises; they are the best possible expression of something not yet consciously recognized. Depending on the dreamer and the context, a phallic symbol may be a penis or an indication of creative potential.

The Healing Zone often bestows a symbol pointing the way to a new myth for your life. The word "symbol" derives from the ancient Greek word *sumballen,* which described the custom of breaking a clay slate and giving a piece to each member of a group before they dispersed. When the group reconvened, the pieces were reassembled—*sumballen* means "to throw together." Through this custom, an individual's group identity was confirmed within the whole—like a piece of a jigsaw puzzle.

A symbol is an unconsciously chosen expression of a latent code (Bedi, 2007), the best possible conscious manifestation of a fact whose existence is sensed. Symbols are pregnant with meaning, and the symbolic value of an expression is contingent upon the attitude of the observing consciousness. Symbols have life-giving and life-enhancing value. They evoke deep emotion and a sense of the numinous. They fascinate, and have a sense of mystery and intrigue. They manifest in a synchronistic matrix and feel relevant to the present situation and emerging trajectory of our lives. Symbols combine many diverse elements into a unitary expression; they tolerate paradox and are emotionally resonant.

In conventional language, symbols are often confused with signs. Although signs and symbols are often interchanged in daily usage, however, they have specific meanings in the literature of analytical psychology. A sign is a representation of something known; it conveys specific information. A sign is expressed in words; it represents logical thinking. A symbol represents fantasy and imaginal thinking. Signs use numerous words to deal with one thought, while one symbolic image may represent the vast mystery of the Healing Zone. A symbol is activated when the underlying archetype is invoked at a time of crisis or trauma, and at developmental and initiatory transitions.

Symbols have two poles—the personal, based on your conscious experience, and the collective, planted in the depths of the psyche where it reaches into the archetypal matrix of the collective consciousness. Symbols connect your ego, or consciousness, to the collective psyche, or the wisdom of the universe. This is their transcendent function. A symbol can manifest as a daydream, a fantasy, a dream, a synchronistic event, a medical or psychiatric illness, a personality hang-up, or a fascinating relationship. They can also be experienced in encounters with art, film, a favorite fairy tale, or even the drawing you doodle when daydreaming.

Another important dimension of Jungian psychology is the theory that dreams can point to the future. They have a Janus quality, like the Greek god with two faces who lent his name to January, the month that bids farewell to the past year and welcomes the year ahead. Teleological dreams learn from the past and beckon the future, laying out the goals of healing.

As Jung pointed out, dreams typically have a recognizable dramatic structure. Much like a film or a novel, they have a setting, plot development, a turning point, and a resolution. Sometimes one or more of these elements is missing, in which case the dream is unfinished. (Don't worry; from time to time, we all have dreams that are or seem incomplete. We can still work with what we have.)

When familiar people and places appear in a dream, they refer to the actual people and places, but also probably to something in your unconscious that resembles those people and places. For example, when your mother or father appears in a dream, the message may be about the mothering or fathering capacity in you. When familiar people or places appear in a dream in ways that differ from reality—age, looks, actions, attitude—you can be pretty sure that the dream is talking about a part of your psyche that functions as those people or places do.

Dreams do not tell you what to do; rather, they provide a different view that may augment, modify, correct, complete, or contradict your conscious position. As a rule, when a dream presents an extreme view of a situation, it is counterbalancing an equal but opposite extreme conscious position. In other words, the truth lies somewhere in the middle.

Working with your own dreams is challenging, because they show you to yourself from a perspective that you do not consciously see. In other words, your dreams fill in your blind spots. That is why it is often expedient to work individually or in a group with a therapist or analyst skilled in dream work. Your dreams can tell you a lot more than you know. Other people will often see meaning in them where you see nothing but the images themselves. Take care that the person to whom you tell your dreams is trustworthy and bears you no ill will. In telling your dreams, you are exposing to the view of others sides of yourself that even you don't see.

Working on your own dreams is about *process*, not *outcome*. It's amazing. The "product" you end up with may not look like much, but the process you have engaged in works on you, and will subtly deepen your consciousness and inform it of the intentions of your soul. With practice, you can master the basic elements of dream work.

I once dreamed of driving a huge, gray garbage truck to deliver food for my wife's catering business. I asked her why we needed such a big truck—wouldn't a small, yellow delivery van with her restaurant's logo on the side be more practical and functional? The plot turned when a close friend and mentor visited us from England. In the dream, he and I took this garbage truck for a ride. To my amazement, he said that he had had a one-day lesson in how to use this truck as an amphibious vessel. We sailed to a small island with our families, and spent a day picnicking on the beach. We stayed at a small condo with a magnificent view of our city. I realized that this was no ordinary truck, and that I needed some brief instruction to explore its amphibian wonders.

The dream showed me that, consciously, I had been trying to simplify my life, transforming it into something like the elegant little yellow delivery van—but it always got complicated and burdensome, like the large gray garbage truck. The dream helped me accept the cumbersome complexities of my life, including acceptance of my wife's restaurant business. I honored my spiritual calling by navigating this truck onto the waters of my unconscious and got a view of life from outside—from island to mainland. I relinquished my wish to be conventional. Paradoxically, accepting my karma of complexity in my life actually started to make my dharmic pursuit simpler. To honor the dream, I went to a toy store that weekend and bought a yellow delivery van and a huge gray garbage truck. They now stand side-by-side in my study.

The dream instructed me about my own Healing Zone. My life was not going to be quaint and simple; I must honor its cumbersome, chaotic complexity and keep cleaning it up regularly with the help of the garbage truck! This truck was an amphibious vessel that could navigate both land and water. As a psychoanalyst, I must engage the challenges of the conscious outer life symbolized by land, yet stay reflective about the mysteries of the unconscious life and the waters of the psyche.

Catching Your Dreams

Patients and students often ask me how best to remember their dreams. Here are some guidelines:

- Go to sleep with the intention of remembering dreams when you awaken. When you go to sleep, suggest to yourself that you will recall a dream *and* that you will write it down.
- Sleep until you wake up naturally; REM sleep has the tendency to wake you up in the last third of the night.
- Establish a dream anchor, a consistent object, as a reminder of your dreams.
- Once awake, lie still, and do not open your eyes until you attend to the dream image in your mind.
- Rehearse the recalled images and give a title to your dream, making recall easier.
- Keep a dream notebook or tape recorder next to your bed. Write down or tape record your dream as soon as you awaken, before getting out of bed.
- On weekends, you can practice dream recall by setting an early alarm, which hopefully will awaken you from a dream and allow you to go back to sleep again!

Working with Your Dreams

- Re-visualize the images of the dream and feel the emotions again. You must re-experience the dream to bring it back to life.
- Consider the structure of your dream. Does it have a setting? Does the action develop? Is there a turning point? Does it reach a conclusion? Dreams often end before the turning point or before they reach a conclusion, which implies that the development cannot go further at that time.
- Contemplate each image. Note the feelings, memories, and impressions that arise when you contemplate each image, situation, or person in the dream. *Stay with the image; circle*

around it; don't let your associations lead you far afield. What does the dream appear to be saying about your life or relationships? What does it tell you about how you get around in the world? How does it portray the emotional and mental space you inhabit? Does it seem to depict what is opposing you or what is assisting you?

- Compare current dreams with other dreams in which the same or similar persons, places, themes, or images have appeared. What changes do you notice? How is your presence in the dream now different than it was in the past?

- After working on a dream, note how your emotional state has changed in the course of your dream work. Note the dream's prescription for your present life dilemma.

- Explore how the dream modifies your conscious assessment of your present life situation and assess its guidance about your future course of action.

- Honor your dream by carrying out some action or ritual in your waking life that pays respect to its images and intent. For example, if a long-forgotten friend appears in your dream, first understand what aspect or quality of this friend you need to activate in your life to deal with a current situation. Then pick up the phone and call your friend. If you honor your dreams and their images with some sacred ritual, they will honor and reward you by continuing to send helpful, guiding messages. These rituals can help to establish a positive feedback loop.

Leveraging the Synchronicity of Dreams

Dreams are always examples of synchronicity, because we always get the right dreams at the right time. One way to think about synchronistic events is to call them meaningful coincidences. A synchronicity may be as simple as dreaming about people you haven't seen in months, then receiving a postcard from them the next morning. It may be the experience of similar or identical thoughts, ideas, or dreams at the same time by different people in different places. Synchronistic events are evidence of a close connection between the parties or things involved. They cannot be explained by causality. They are a kind of "heads up" that urges you to pay attention.

Your soul arranges synchronistic events to draw your attention to energies, events, people, and circumstances. When cosmic forces, your soul energy, and events and people in your outer life are in optimal alignment, it is a mysterious and sacred moment that allows some invisible aspect of your soul to become visible, if only you acknowledge it, attend to it, and act upon it in a conscious manner.

I once decided to meet a colleague to discuss a research idea. Given our busy schedules, we both decided to have a brown-bag meeting. To our amazement, we found that both of us had, independently, packed a grilled chicken sandwich on whole wheat bread with a dill pickle and bags of potato chips of identical size. Immediately, I knew that our souls had spoken and that the outcome of our cooperation would be numinous. We co-authored an excellent article that was published in a reputable journal, received broad acclaim, and made a small but significant contribution to improving a certain treatment method. This synchronistic event activated the latent code of twin-ship and collaboration.

Active Imagination

Active imagination is a method of personifying the unconscious. It creates a bridge between the consciousness and a selected aspect of the unconscious. The starting point of active imagination can be a dream image, a mood, or any spontaneous visual image. Von Franz was the first to describe the four stages involved in the active imagination (see figure 15). Other eminent Jungians, including Reverend Robert Johnson (Johnson, 1989) and Barbara Hannah (Hannah, 1999), made significant contributions to the project. For them, active imagination is a conscious attempt to modify and temporarily suspend the ego complex to accentuate the faint whisper of the unconscious in the sacred realm of consciousness.

In active imagination, you take a product of the unconscious—a mood or a dream image, a creative artifact, a medical or psychiatric symptom, a relationship tangle or a synchronistic event—and explore your ego's experience of this fractal of your soul. Once the soul fractal and its waking ego experience are held together under the observing consciousness, this consciousness activates the Healing Zone, which moves you from illness to wellness (Von Franz, 1997).

Active imagination relies on four stages:

- Engaging the unconscious
- Imagining a dialogue between the conscious ego and a personified part of the unconscious
- Embodying the soul symbol
- Precipitating an ethical confrontation between the ego and the soul

The first stage involves several layers of engagement with the unconscious. To begin, you must empty your mind of the ego's many trains of thought—your restless "monkey mind"—and allow images from the unconscious to surface and make contact with your conscious mind. Closing your eyes and focusing on your breath as you gradually relax your body can help to quiet your monkey mind and shift your consciousness from logical thinking to archaic, primitive, or primary-process (imaginal, non-rational) thinking. Here, ego plays the role of the conscious recorder—the scribe of the soul.

My patient John, whom we met before, complained of feeling sad, moody, and depressed. I invited him to personify this feeling. Gradually, his feeling took the form of his aunt, Mita, to whom he was close as a child. Diagnosed as an attention-deficit hyperactive

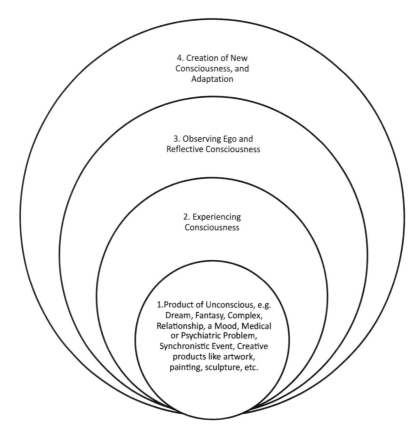

Figure 15. The four stages of active imagination.

child, John often went to Mita's home after school. She was an island of serenity in his otherwise chaotic life, a symbol of calm and sacred space. Because of his personality and hyperactivity disorder, John confused serenity with depression and boredom. Gradually, he was able to reclaim this island of tranquility within his sea of emotional chaos.

Once you have engaged your unconscious, an imagined dialogue between your conscious ego and a personified part of the unconscious emerges. It may be an auditory event in which the voice of your unconscious is heard in response to questions. Other modes of dialogue with the unconscious include painting, sculpting, movement, dancing, or writing. John's dialogue with his long-dead aunt took written form.

Dialogue between ego and soul is not enough, however. For the process to be complete, your ego must react to what has been expressed in its conversation with your unconscious, then draw conclusions and put them to work in your life. Jung emphasized the importance of concretizing the work to prevent its content from slipping back into the unconscious. Jung's own encounter with the unconscious using active imagination is embodied in his posthumously published personal diary, *The Red Book*, which is a valuable guide to those aspiring to use this method (Jung, 2009).

To establish this dialogue, you should use a secondary or undeveloped talent. For example, a writer may paint or sculpt; a painter may dance. The danger in using a familiar talent is that skill serves the ego rather than expressing the unconscious. The mistakes that surface when treading on unfamiliar ground express your unconscious and interfere with your ego's intentions. Mistakes are the cracks in consciousness through which Aditi whispers the intentions of your soul.

Next, you must work and rework the material into a creative formulation that will inevitably be in accord with your aesthetic taste or artistic sense. Then you must invoke the ego's understanding to comprehend the meaning of the unconscious product. Your true essence is revealed by how your ego interacts with the unconscious product or images that surface through active imagination. The danger is that you may feel that the product is nothing but art. In fact, the image must be treated as if it were as real as anything in the material world for it to have a healing influence on your psyche. Jung painted and sculpted his fantasies, but took care to amplify those images through his understanding of myth and alchemy. Creative formulation engages your body in the work, forming a bridge between the worlds of Spirit and matter.

John's continuing dialogue with the image of his favorite aunt was not enough to alleviate his depression. The dialogue had to be embodied and lived out, which happened when he started making room for sacred space in his driven, mundane life. This included silence, solitude, studio time, journaling, prayer and meditation, playing golf, and just staying home two evenings a week.

Now, the ego needs to have it out with the unconscious. A democracy must be established between the ego and the unconscious, with both entities having an equal vote. This may entail a long conflict between them, and may eventually demand sacrifices from both sides.

Von Franz recommends the following guidelines for dealing with the creative formulation from the unconscious. First, apply the image of active imagination to ordinary life. Show love, devotion, and respect for the unconscious by acknowledging it, communicating with it often, and integrating images and insights gained into life and consciousness. Von Franz warns, however, that something physical must be performed to decrease the risk of intellectualization. Likewise, Robert Johnson emphasizes the need to ritualize the insight within a day or two of its surfacing. The performance of some ritual— a symbolic behavior consciously performed—honors the image from the unconscious and gives it substance.

There are clinical benefits to invoking active imagination. In therapy, patients whose dreams seldom have form or structure may be burdened with an unconscious that is overflowing, bursting at the seams. Rather than let this unconscious "abscess" burst, therapists may pierce it and drain it consciously through active imagination. Conversely, they may apply active imagination when patients have too few dreams. For other individuals, an impenetrable complex or life problem may be the focus of active imagination. If they continually make the same errors, it can be helpful for them to personify their root complexes through active imagination.

Active imagination is not helpful for schizophrenics, because they are already living in the soul. They are on the other side. In their case, they must build their ego complexes by strengthening their external adaptation. British psychiatrist Maxwell Jones proposes creating a container for psychotic or schizophrenic patients who lack either an ego container to hold the unconscious or a solid bridge to the unconscious. In such cases, a bridge or solid structure of containment must be built by a tight therapeutic program. This may entail group therapy—sometimes even several times a day. For Maxwell Jones, the group itself becomes the skin or the shell of the patient.

That is one technique. Another is the use of medications, which become a protective shell around the unconscious. What medications really do is mediate—like the red lights on the merging lanes on a freeway. They regulate how much of the unconscious is able to join the freeway of ego consciousness. Establishing a structure is the key for very sick patients. Structure can also be created through therapy involving sculpting, dancing, and art, which give new venues in which the unconscious can speak, so that it does not always have to voice itself through the psychosis.

Engaging the Active Imagination

- Start with a dream image, a mood, or any spontaneous visual image. This must relate to some problem, tangle, crisis, or issue you are presently confronting.
- Center yourself by letting go of your "monkey mind"—all mental distractions—so that you can focus on your inquiry. Find a quiet, solitary place to proceed where you will be free of interruptions, phone calls, etc. for up to an hour.
- Close your mind for a while and breathe with intention and rhythm to deepen your consciousness.
- Let your regular consciousness become just an observer or witness to the rest of the process. It may become a scribe or recorder.
- Invite the image or the mood to take a form. If it refuses, assign it a form.
- Decide how you will have a dialogue with this image. Will you write it? Draw it? Express it in dance movement? For best

results, use an inferior function as a medium of dialogue. For example, a writer may paint or sculpt; a painter may dance, etc.

- Treat the image with which you have chosen to dialogue as you would in real life, showing it devotion and respect. If the image suggests something that is not viable in real life, challenge it. If it suggests something that is reasonable but difficult to implement, resolve to do it.
- Implement the decided intervention based on your dialogue within the next twenty-four hours.
- Journal how this image affects you emotionally.
- Maintain a sense of aesthetics and respect in your dialogue. For instance, if you are writing the dialogue, do it with deliberation. If you are drawing your response, make it the most aesthetic drawing that you possibly can.

Fascinations and Antipathies

Whenever you experience fascination or antipathy, you are reacting to a reflection of some part of your Healing Zone that is not adequately integrated into your conscious personality. Attraction tells you that you want what you see; repulsion tells you the opposite. Either way, your soul is reacting to a reflection of its unlived potential. For one reason or another, this unlived potential has not been ennobled in your lived life.

Fascinations and antipathies are signals from the soul that the present situation offers optimal conditions for the incarnation of this potential. You do not fully control fascinations or antipathies, attractions or repulsions, since they emanate from the depths of your soul rather than your waking consciousness. They can be in response to another person, an idea, a potential experience, or a memory. The list is nearly inexhaustible.

Dan is a surgeon in his forties who consulted me for depression in the midst of his divorce. He reported that he was a very inartistic, left-brain individual with little interest in art, literature, and the lighter side of life. He was disturbed to find himself aimlessly wandering in the evenings, invariably ending up at a toyshop and gazing into the window at science toys with no conscious interest in anything in particular. He worried that this was some kind of obsession. I invited him to honor this fascination rather than be critical of it, asking how he could see the science toys fitting into his life.

What surfaced in our discussion was that Dan was unconsciously fascinated by and consciously antipathetic to telescopes. An interest in astronomy was a childhood dream of Dan's that was strongly discouraged by his physician father, who wanted his son to follow in his footsteps. I proposed that he needed to honor this repressed interest in astronomy in some way, perhaps by taking classes at the local university. Dan undertook this enterprise mostly to placate me. I am happy to report that he is now an adept amateur astronomer. He uses a special computerized telescope and has received considerable acclaim for his blossoming talent. Astronomy now embodies both the emotional and aesthetic aspects of Dan's soul. In getting in touch with the finer aspects of his soulfulness, he has been able to repair his marriage. A fascination with the stars put him in touch with the Healing Zone to engage his creative psyche.

Our relationships benefit when we attend to the Healing Zone. Close relationships bring out the best and worst in us and can be a crucible in which we are transformed by the fire of intense emotions. The old saying, "opposites attract," is often true. When you are attracted to someone who seems to be your missing half, you are really attracted to a part of you that is lacking. In fact, this "missing half" is usually a part of you that is difficult to develop and often at odds with a more developed facet of your personality. After the initial "honeymoon phase" of these relationships, you may experience disappointment and disillusionment, as you discover that "the other" is not entirely as you thought. This realization tells you that you were seeing only part of the other person—the part that was your own unknown face reflected back to you—a face that made you feel complete.

An overwhelming attraction is strong evidence that you are experiencing another person as an opposite to yourself. Although you may not recognize it at the time, an overwhelming attraction is a measure of the gulf between you and the other person, but also of the gulf between your conscious view of yourself and your unlived soul—as well as the amount of energy needed to bridge that gulf. When you learn how to deal with both difficult and attractive aspects of relationships, you have the opportunity to access and cultivate a facet of your soul that you see in that other person.

Work out a plan of action to develop your inferior skills and abilities that were hitherto carried by your partner. Monitor your progress to see how much of what was carried by the other person is now managed by you, using your own skills and potentials.

Rachel and Steve have been married for two years. Steve is a quiet, caring, devoted husband—an engineer by trade. Rachel is a vivacious, beautiful, attention-seeking hysteric. When they went to a bar, she socialized effervescently with other men, often got drunk, and wanted to stay till the wee hours of the morning, while Steve got tired and insisted on leaving early to be prepared for work the following day.

Rachel's father abandoned her mother when she was pregnant with Rachel, so she never met him, nor has she ever seen his picture. Consciously, she found strength and security in Steve's rock-solid personality. Unconsciously, however, she kept provoking him. On closer exploration of their relationship, it became apparent that she had a hostile-dependent attachment to Steve. She attempted to reincarnate her missing father through him, provoking him to set limits on her as if he were her parent and simultaneously behaving in a provocative and contemptuous manner to metabolize her rage at an abandoning father.

I invited Rachel to explore what she would do if Steve left after offering to take her home and agreeing to come and pick her up from the bar whenever she was ready. She commented that she would be enraged and get drunk just to get even with him. I deepened this image. She reported that she would get drunk several times and be there till six in the morning, hoping that Steve would call and come looking for her. "What if he didn't?" I inquired. "Then reluctantly I'd call my friend Mary to come pick me up," she replied. I exclaimed: "So finally, you would take care of yourself!" Rachel was amused and amazed that she could parent herself, and did not need to project this need for a father onto her loving husband all the time.

This is one vignette from a multitude of similar interventions that gradually helped Rachel recognize that what she sought in her marriage was a father who would take care of her and with whom she could retire her anger at her biological father for abandoning her. Gradually, she learned to parent herself, unburdening her marriage of the dynamic of hostile dependency. Her own capacity to be her own good parent and a loving wife was reincarnated in the sacred vessel of the marriage. Her hostile dependency on her husband became the channel through which Rachel could activate the latent code of her soul to engage the archetype of Father within— the missing father she had projected onto her husband all her married life.

Steve had always wanted to be a playful, carefree Bohemian person, but his rough-and-tumble childhood with an alcoholic father and a depressed mother did not permit such a luxury. He projected his desire for a Bohemian life onto Rachel, who lived it out in a hysterical lifestyle. As Rachel took ownership of her self-parenting, Steve gradually started to relinquish his heroic adaptation and made room for the more laid-back, relaxed, and playful aspects of his soul.

Exploring Your Fascinations and Antipathies

- Carefully note the content and the emotions you experience. Every detail may be significant, so do not edit and do not elaborate (yet). Get the facts.
- Systematically review the content and emotion of the experience. For each image in the content, and for each emotion, note down what spontaneously comes to mind.
- Consider of what or of whom the image reminds you. Where or with whom have you felt these emotions?
- Ask yourself what was or is the significance of the image or emotion. What role did the image or emotion play in your life in the past?
- Consider what role the image or emotion plays now.
- If you are exploring a fascination, identify what it is in the content of the fascination that you want as a part of yourself. How would incorporating the content of the fascination change your life now?
- If you are exploring an antipathy, identify what it is in the content of the antipathy that you want to disown. How would eliminating the content of the antipathy change your life now?
- List and prioritize the steps you can take to effect the changes you have identified.
- Be sure to chart your progress.

Complexes and Hang-ups

Complexes are a normal part of our psychological make-up. Not all complexes are troublesome, but problem complexes are the ones that we most often notice. Your complexes are your emotionally vulnerable spots. You "go ballistic" or "fly off the handle" when someone triggers a volatile complex by word or deed.

Complexes take shape around typical human experiences—birth, death, marriage, transitions, parents, siblings, etc. The core pattern of a complex is archetypal (that is, typically human, and not a personal acquisition). The specific content, or shell, of a complex, however, derives from your life experience. Together, core and shell constitute the whole complex.

Complexes manifest in several ways. Perhaps the most frequent are found in your relationships (as fascinations, antipathies, and other strong emotional reactions), in spontaneous discharges of strong emotion, and in dreams and fantasies. When a complex is activated, your behavior changes in four ways: your adaptation regresses to that of an earlier developmental level; you become more emotional; you blame another for "making" you react; and your emotions tend to rumble about in you for a long time. Learning to understand your soul's messages sent in the form of activated complexes offers you a steppingstone to fuller actualization of your latent code.

Because of relationship problems with her peers, Trudy's employer referred her to me for treatment. In her first session, Trudy, a mid-level executive, took control and spoke incessantly, giving me little opportunity to ask questions. When this pattern continued for a few sessions, I confronted her. She broke down in remorse and tears, and fell into a long silence. When I invited her to share the image in her mind, she recalled an incident on Christmas Eve when she was eight years old.

Trudy's father was drunk and watching TV; her mother was depressed and had retreated to her bedroom. Her two oldest siblings were trying to manage the household; the younger children were in chaos. Trudy remembered darting first to her father's room and then to her mother's, chattering incessantly as she tried to revive them from their alcoholic and depressive stupors above the din of the chaotic family.

Trudy's anxious, excited manner of speaking began as a way to resuscitate her emotionally dead parents. This became an intrusive, overbearing complex that was triggered regularly in staff meetings at work. Through a long process of analysis, Trudy learned to honor and hold her anxiety and to hear others out. People began to seek out her views and opinions with respect. As a result, she steadily climbed the corporate ladder and made substantial contributions to the success of her enterprise. Her overbearing complex offered her a path to the Healing Zone. When she worked out the child-hood dynamic that created this complex, she was able to claim her authentic authority, resulting in well-deserved affirmation at work and in her personal life.

Over decades of clinical practice as a psychiatrist and Jung-ian psychoanalyst, I have surmised that, when all is said and done, there are two groups of individuals who seek psychotherapy. The first suffers from a God complex. These individuals have an inflated sense of themselves. They take themselves too seriously, consider themselves the center of the universe, and have an inflated sense of self-esteem. They believe that the world revolves around them and assume that their worldview is the only lens through which reality can be perceived. They see other people as mere mirrors that must reflect their own grandeur and must only speak to echo their pro-nouncements.

Individuals with a God complex see their personal and pro-fessional relationships as an extension of their wondrous selves; any attempt by others to assert an opposing viewpoint is met with surprise, disdain, and retaliation. They choose spouses with low self-esteem who can be molded easily. Their children are groomed to become ambassadors of their grand mission, without any chance for healthy self-assertion—until, of course, they are old enough to protest and rebel through acting out, drug addiction, or other meth-ods of resistance. In therapy, they always get into power struggles with their therapists who, in their view, fail to understand their true value or worth. They may go doctor shopping to find a therapist who appreciates how special they are.

The second group seeking psychotherapy has a dog complex—a depleted sense of self-esteem. They stay at the margins of their families or professions and tend to avoid attention. They underachieve in their professional lives and permit themselves to be treated as doormats in personal relationships. They are attracted to individuals with a God complex in order to bask in their reflected glory. They live off the emotional crumbs of these powerful individuals and underplay their own ideas or potential contributions to their personal growth, their families, and their communities. They are drawn to one powerful person after another and are attracted to new movements, cults, or therapists who happen to be in vogue, rather than undertaking the serious journey from illness to wellness.

It is interesting that both groups are usually caught in relationships with the other. The God complex needs the dog complex to worship it. The dog complex needs the God complex to redeem it. These opposites attract each other. The alliance works very well during the honeymoon phase of a relationship, but when these mutual projections cannot be sustained, the relationship begins to sour. When the God individuals cannot sustain their godliness because they hit the hard rock of reality, they seek therapy because the world does not appreciate their true worth. They come to therapy to lick their wounded dreams of glory and success. Confronted by the reality of aging, illness, and disappointment, they want to change the mirror rather than reflect on their own situations. They seek medications to boost their flagging self-esteem rather than undertake a soul-searching reevaluation of their predicament. They often change jobs or partners until they find mirrors that distort their reality to fit their grandiose view of themselves. This is a temporary fix that will soon break down.

The dog people need powerful others to hold and sustain them at the cost of sacrificing their authentic potential. They end up in clingy, codependent relationships with God people. These alliances start breaking down when their souls push for maturation and self-assertion, and move from the dynamic of self-concealment to self-revelation. A seed cannot stay dormant in the soil forever, just as a tree cannot grow into the sky immediately. Nature and the psyche have their own rhythms. There is a time to be dormant and a time to blossom, even for someone with a dog complex. There are trees that blossom even beside the concrete freeways where soil is limited. The soul always finds a way to incarnate into consciousness.

The dance between the dog complex and the God complex plays out in seven types of personality maturation and relationship development: Victim/Aggressor, Exploiter/Martyr, Master/Slave, Caretaker/Codependent, Intimidator/Silent One, Leader/Follower, and Narcissist/Autistic. Through psychotherapy, these relationship splits can be recognized and brought to the surface. Their projections can be worked through and the authentic core personality can be given an opportunity to emerge and blossom. God-complex individuals have to honor their inner dog with humility and attention—their unlived vulnerable aspects, their shadow side, their underdeveloped aspects—for example, the feeling function for intellectuals and the sensate function for intuitive types.

Those who suffer from the dog complex start to heal when they acknowledge their unlived and unacknowledged skills, strengths, and potentials on the stage of consciousness and lived life. They learn to assert themselves in relationships, honor their creative side, find their own voices, refuse to permit self-victimization, and stake out their own ground in personal and professional encounters. They reclaim the lost continent of their souls. When you heal the God/dog split in yourself and live your life with humility, but also in celebration of your creative potentials—when you are able to laugh at yourself, but also make your substantial and worthy dharmic contribution to the welfare of your soul, your family, your community, and your world—you become whole and heal the inner wounds of your soul. That is a well-lived life.

Recognizing Your Complexes

- Define what you mean by a complex.
- List the important complexes in your life. What emotions does each one provoke—e.g., sadness, joy, anger, fear.

- Consider what happens in your body when a complex is activated.
- Identify the person who is routinely implicated as messing up your day or plans when a complex is triggered.
- Identify each important person or event in your life that contributed to this complex—e.g., father, mother, grandparent, immigration, school, illness, etc.
- Describe the impact that each complex has had on your life in the past and the present.
- Consider the individuals, events, and circumstances that activate your complexes.

Retiring Your Complexes

How do we retire complexes? That is, how do you recognize the complex and challenge old behaviors and assumptions about yourself, the world, and the future? How do you experiment with new behaviors, and remain open to let help arrive from friends, family, therapists, or others?

- Start by recognizing when you have become unusually emotional.
- Identify the trigger event that activated your emotions (in case it is not obvious).
- Identify and note down your emotions, your fantasies, and your memories of similar experiences (people, places, events).
- Consider what unresolved issue or undeveloped potential is represented by the complex.
- Assess how effective your usual way of dealing with the activated complex is.
- Work out a sequence of different behaviors (in increasing order of difficulty) to address the core issue in the complex.
- Chart your progress by noting habits and behaviors contrary to your own nature when situations and individuals activate your

complex. This results in increased lead time, more rapid recovery from the effects of your complex, and less frequent activation.

Cognitive Distortions

One of the crucial tasks in engaging the present moment rather than remaining in the past or wandering off into the future is to clean the lens through which you perceive yourself, others, and the world. Your lens may be clouded by cognitive distortions (Beck 1980; 1979) based on past experiences and psychological wounds associated with significant individuals in your environment—for example, your parents.

The most common cognitive distortions are:

- **All-or-nothing thinking**: Considering everything in absolute terms—e.g., "always," "every," or "never." Few aspects of human behavior are so absolute.
- **Overgeneralization**: Using isolated cases to make wide generalizations.
- **Mental filters**: Focusing exclusively on certain, usually negative or upsetting, aspects while ignoring the rest.
- **Disqualifying the positive**: Continually "shooting down" positive experiences for arbitrary reasons.
- **Jumping to conclusions**: Assuming something negative where there is no evidence to support it. Two specific subtypes are mind-reading—assuming the intentions of others—and fortune-telling—predicting how things will turn out before they happen.
- **Magnification and minimization**: Understating or exaggerating people or situations. Often, positive characteristics are exaggerated and negative characteristics understated. A

subtype of magnification, catastrophizing, focuses on the worst possible outcome, however unlikely. A catastrophizer deems a situation unbearable or impossible when it is really just uncomfortable.

- **Emotional reasoning**: Making decisions and arguments based on feelings rather than objective reality.
- **"Should" statements**: Concentrating on what you think "should" or ought to be rather than the actual situation confronting you. When you make "should" statements, you try to apply rigid rules, no matter what the circumstances.
- **Labeling**: Explaining behaviors or events merely by naming them, rather than describing specifics. When you assign a label to others (or yourself), you lock them in absolute and unalterable terms.
- **Personalization**: Assuming you or others directly caused things when that may not have been the case. When applied to others, this is an example of blame.

Here are some of the realizations I have found clinically and personally helpful in dealing with cognitive distortions or the dance of the monkey mind.

- A distorted perceptual lens leads to faulty evaluation of yourself, others, and the future.
- A distorted lens causes inaccurate feelings, including anger, sadness, fear, guilt, and shame.
- These feelings are based on the distortion that the present situation, with its associated thoughts and feelings, is permanent and not transient.
- We attempt to hang on to situations, thoughts, and feelings that create a temporary illusion of pleasure; we try to avoid others in a misguided attempt to avoid pain. Both attempts lead to suffering, since they avoid reflecting on the deeper aspect of pres-

ent reality. When we do this, we are just rearranging the deck chairs on the Titanic.

- Distorted feelings lead to inner and relationship turbulence, activating cravings for alcohol, drugs, food, sex, gambling, and pornography. They can also lead to regression to old symptoms to establish an illusion of safety. This may take the form of compulsions, panic, anxiety, headaches, backache, and neck pain.
- Replace your cognitive distortions with rational, viable alternative explanations, reasonable alternative thoughts, sober choices, and reflective actions in the given situation.

Centering Prayer

Centering prayer is a useful method to hold your waking ego in conscious juxtaposition to your bliss body and your soul. This creates a holding vessel to receive the grace and the gift of the divine to heal your mind, body, and soul. Based on the meditative practices of the East that have been creatively amplified in recent times by the Roman Catholic Benedictine order, centering prayer places a strong emphasis on interior silence. It consists of the following steps (Pennington, 1982; Keating, 2009):

- Sit comfortably with your eyes closed. Relax and quiet yourself. Be in love with the divine.
- Choose a sacred word that best supports your intention to be in the divine presence and open to its action within you (i.e., "peace," "spirit," "love").
- Let that word be gently present as a symbol of your sincere intention to be in the divine presence. When any other thoughts, feelings, perceptions, images, or associations come to mind, simply return to your sacred word as if it were your anchor.

Chapter 4

Accessing the Healing Zone

Now that you understand how your brain, your ego, and your soul engage with the Healing Zone, you are ready to access it using any one of a number of methods that have come to us from a variety of traditions and cultures. These include yoga, breath control, meditation, mindfulness, music, mandala and yantra therapy, and Kundalini balancing.

Yoga

Yoga is an ancient healing and spiritual practice based on exercises for the physical body. *Yoga* means "to yoke"—by extension, to bind the ego to the soul and the soul to Spirit. It yokes personal consciousness to universal consciousness through a variety of disciplines or paths. Gyana yoga, or yoga through knowledge, includes the study of the psyche and Spirit. It may embrace psychoanalysis, philosophy, and the Talmudic tradition. Bhakti yoga unites you with the divine via love and devotion; it appeals to those who choose the path of faith as the way to God. Bhakti yoga corresponds to the work of Mother Teresa and much of the Christian spiritual tradition. Karma yoga binds you to the divine by encouraging you to live your life in tune with your dharma or spiritual calling. Mahatma Gandhi embodied the path of karma yoga, which is built on the cornerstone of simple living and high thinking. It is the preferred path for intuitive individuals.

Hatha yoga focuses on mastery of the body to access the Healing Zone. It can take the route of *asanas,* or body-posture control, and *pranayama,* or breath control, whose true purpose is less to

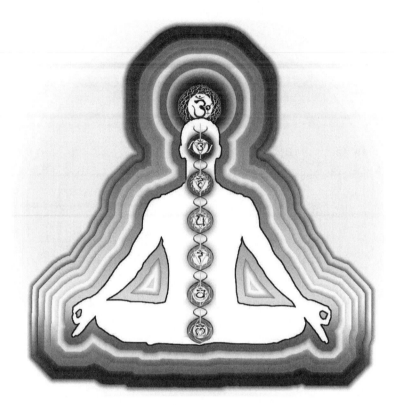

Figure 16. The eight preparatory steps on the path to yoga.
See also Plate 1, color insert following page 160.

train the body than to steady the mind and make the body fit to engage Spirit (Iyengar, 1985, 2001). Hatha yoga is the most popular yoga in the West.

Hindu scriptures outline the eight preparatory steps on the path to yoga (see figure 16 above and color insert Plate 1):

- *Yama*—universal moral commandments
- *Niyama*—self-purification
- *Asana*—body postures
- *Pranayama*—breath management
- *Pratyahara*—withdrawal of consciousness from external senses

- *Dharana*—concentration
- *Dhayna*—meditation
- *Samadhi*—the state of super-consciousness or bliss

The physical body is a temple of the soul. Yoga honors the physical body as a vehicle for the Healing Zone. When all other whispers fail, your soul will send you distress signals in the form of physical illness. When you decipher those signals as symbols of your soul's attempt to guide you back to emotional and spiritual health, the symptoms can abate. You must attend to your body and posture with mindfulness.

The word *pranayama* is a Sanskrit compound of the words *prana*, or "life force," and *yama*, or "death force." The word suggests our need to govern the life and death forces in the psyche. This is accomplished by breath control. On average, each of us breathes 23,000 times a day. We take about 600 million breaths during a lifetime. You can live without food for as long as forty days and without water for seven. You can survive only six to eight minutes without air. Breath (*pnuema*) is seen as a gift of Spirit in many traditions. Hindus believe that each breath, when engaged meditatively, is an invocation of the divine Spirit that yokes us to the numinous or the divine in the universe.

Pranayama is an essential component of the practice of yoga for centering the consciousness. Prana, or life energy, is the gift of the universe that sustains us in this lifetime. When we die physically, our life energy merges with the cosmic, or collective, energy. At this point of transition, the Atman (individual consciousness) merges with the Brahman (divine consciousness). We return to the Source.

While the most immediate manifestation of prana is the breath, ancient Indian texts classify five different types of vital energy, or *prana vayus*—*prana, apana, samana, udana*, and *vyana*. These are specific manifestations of the general life energy or vital wind (*pneuma*). Prana vayu controls the breathing in the thoracic region.

Apana vayu moves in the lower abdomen and controls the elimination of urine, semen, and feces. Samana vayu regulates the gastric processes aiding digestion. Udana vayu operates in the throat (the pharynx and larynx) and regulates the vocal cords and the intake of food and air. Vyana vayu is a body-wide system of energy distribution or metabolism that distributes energy derived from food and breath through the circulatory system, while removing toxins and metabolic waste. In pranayama, inhalation and the apana vayu activate the prana vayu by exhalation. Vyana vayu acts as mediator of prana and apana vayus by distributing energy and removing toxic metabolites. The visible expression of this complex vital life energy in your consciousness is the movement of your lungs in respiration.

Normally, prana (breath) is in constant association with consciousness, which is usually driven by desire. If you can steady your prana, you can center your consciousness and free it from desire. This freedom permits you to move from sexual and other mundane ego desires to the spiritual realm of consciousness. When your energy body is centered, it steadies all the other koshas, or layers of consciousness, including the physical, emotional, and intellectual bodies. This allows you to move into your bliss body, close to your soul and Spirit—the Atman and the Brahman.

The Indian tradition has perfected the art of prana—breathing with intention, technique, and purpose—through regulating inhalation (puraka), exhalation (rechaka), and retention of breath (kumbhaka). Puraka infuses energy and oxygen into your body. Rechaka eliminates toxins. Kumbhaka is the energy- and toxin-management system of the prana. Pranayama must only be practiced in conjunction with asana, or optimal body postures, so as not to impede the flow of energy. It gives you a valuable tool to master the energy body and to center your consciousness, steadying all the other koshas or sheaths of your consciousness and aligning you to your bliss body, Atman (soul), and the flow of the universe (Spirit).

Pranayama also offers pragmatic dividends (Iyengar, 1985). For instance, when your consciousness is steadied during moderate, guided breath retention, your heart rate slows, enhancing your calming, cooling parasympathetic nervous system as well as resting your heart muscle. This increases longevity. Pranayama can also alleviate pain in your physical body.

Once you are trained in basic pranayama techniques, you must map out your problems by circling the points on your body that are in pain. Next, establish a quiet, sacred meditative environment in a study or bedroom where you can be comfortable. Lie down on a yoga mat or a carpet, or sit up in a comfortable chair with back support. Then establish the rhythm of breath meditation and focus on the problem area of your body. While mentally focusing on this part of your body, continue the breath meditation or the pranayama exercise given below.

With each breath, you will experience a gradual diminution of pain and discomfort. Complete ten breaths while maintaining a passive focus on the problem area or painful part of your body. You may experience a 10 percent reduction in discomfort with every breath you take.

After ten breaths, take five more. The object of your pain or discomfort will become more relaxed with each breath. At the end of the exercise, stay calm and passive for a few more breaths before gradually returning to normal, daily consciousness. To maintain the effect of pranayama on your physical body, continue this practice daily for thirty minutes.

Breathing with Intention

There are many valuable relaxation methods you can use, like the "1–2, 1–2, 1–2, 1–2" technique—a very simple breathing technique based on yogic breathing or *pranayama* (breath-control) principles.

- Sit in a very relaxed posture. Remember that there are two types of breathing: chest breathing (breathing through your rigid rib cage) and tummy breathing (breathing through your flexible abdominal cavity). Breathing through something flexible is more relaxing than breathing through something rigid, so always breathe through your tummy when you want to relax.

- Put your dominant hand—your right hand, if you are right-handed—on your navel. Remember that this is not deep breathing; it is slow breathing. Deep breathing will actually distract you. This exercise is merely to slow your breathing down.

- Inhale slowly, feeling your tummy rise, and hold for two counts. Then gently breathe out to another count of two. Do this ten times.

- As you breathe out each time, focus on the object you have chosen for relaxation. It may be a flower or a crystal or an image or a stone. You can use the word "relax" or "Shanti" (goddess of peace) if you can't find a focus, or if you are in an unfamiliar place or even a hotel room. Just think the word "relax" as you breathe out.

- Ten repetitions of this pattern will center you tremendously. Being in touch with your navel centers you as well, because the navel chakra is the control chakra. Once you are there, you get hold of your consciousness.

- Use this intentional breathing technique for five to ten minutes two or three times a day. You can also use it whenever you're feeling anxious, panicked, or in pain, if you are experiencing an addictive craving, or just to center yourself and get more focused.

Meditation

Meditation is a private religious devotion or mental exercise in which techniques of concentration and contemplation are used to reach a heightened level of spiritual awareness. The practice has existed in all religions since ancient times. In Hinduism, it was systematized in the school of yoga. One aspect of yoga, *dhyana* (Sanskrit for "concentrated meditation"), gave rise to a school of its own among Buddhists and became the basis of Zen.

In many religions, meditation involves verbal or mental repetition of a single syllable, word, or text (mantras), visual images (mandalas), or devices like prayer wheels or rosaries. These can be useful in focusing concentration. In the 20th century, secular movements like transcendental meditation emerged to teach meditation techniques outside a religious context.

There are essentially two forms of meditation: directed meditation, which focuses on a mantra (usually drawn from scripture or the sayings of a teacher), and undirected meditation, which observes whatever floats through consciousness without holding it in focus. Both forms are valuable. Focused meditation disciplines the mind to focus on an object of choice, ignoring all distractions, while undirected meditation disciplines the mind to detach, to let go.

In addition to the eight preparatory steps on the path to yoga mentioned previously, meditation benefits from the following practices:

- **Create a sacred space**: Pick a place that is as private and safe as possible. This may be your study or bedroom, or any quiet place in your home or office.
- **HALT**: Pick a time to practice your meditation when you are least likely to be disturbed. You should not be overly (H)ungry, (A)ngry, (L)onely, or (T)ired—hence the HALT method—or have just finished eating, as these conditions may cause you to be distracted.
- **Visualize a warm light**: Picture yourself in a cocoon of soothing white light. Feel the light as relaxing. Play with this sphere of light, making it bigger or smaller until it feels right for you. Say to yourself: "I am protected by the pure white light of all that is good and truthful. I am surrounded by the pure light that keeps out all unwanted and evil influences."

- **Follow your breath**: Learn to control and pay attention to your breathing. Start by taking a deep breath in through your nose, breathe into your tummy and hold it for a mental count of three, and then let it all out slowly through your mouth. Repeat this until you begin to feel at rest and relaxed.

- **Relax in the light**: As you breathe, see yourself lying in a light that is warm and pleasant to be in. Starting with the tips of your toes, feel the light relaxing all of your body, slowly moving up into your legs, your trunk, and then into your arms and fingers. As you feel this, become more and more relaxed; go deeper and deeper into a calm and quiet place.

- **Invite your focal thought**: When you feel totally relaxed and at peace, bring a single thought into your mind—think of a pleasant experience or of an idea like love, joy, peace, or compassion. Focus on this one thought and, if some other thought tries to intrude, picture it as written on a clear board between you and your focal thought. Then picture it being erased from that board as it might be from a piece of paper. Quickly dispose of any thought other than your focal thought.

- **Concentrate on your thought**: Try to maintain concentration on your focal thought for at least five minutes. Picture it as being real and experience it as if it were. When you are able to do this and can exclude all other thoughts as they attempt to enter your mind, you will have learned the single most important technique of meditation.

- **Reconnect with outer consciousness**: Come back to normal consciousness by slowly letting the thought fade from your mind and again becoming aware of the warm light. As you feel the light bathing you in its relaxing glow, start to reconnect your mind with the physical sensations of your body. Become aware of your breathing and the room around you. Do this slowly and calmly. When you are fully aware of your surroundings, open your eyes slowly. Enjoy the sense of joy, calm, and peace.

The four essential elements for achieving medical benefits from meditation are a quiet environment, a mental device (an object, word, sound, or image), a passive attitude (vital for evoking the relaxation response), and a comfortable position (Benson, 1975). Of these, the most important are maintaining your mental device and a passive attitude.

Just as an electrocardiogram (ECG) measures the electrical activity of the heart, doctors use the electroencephalogram (EEG) to study the electrical activity of the brain. Recent studies in which the brain states of meditators were monitored by EEG show that those practicing undirected or mindful meditation enjoyed a conscious brain rate (called gamma activity) of 24–40 Hz per second or higher, while those practicing directed or concentration meditation relaxed their brains to calm alpha and theta states at rates of 8–12 and 4–8 Hz per second, respectively.

Measurements by EEG indicate an overall slowing of rates in the alpha and theta states subsequent to meditation and related to the proficiency of the individual's meditation practice, while neuroimaging studies indicate an increase in cerebral blood flow during meditation. Taken together, these studies seem to indicate that meditation prompts changes in the anterior cingulate cortex and dorsolateral prefrontal areas of the brain (Lutz, 2004; Cahn, 2006).

Imagine you are suddenly disturbed by a loud noise while reading. If the same sound is repeated a few seconds later, your attention will again be diverted from reading, only not as strongly or for as long a time. If the noise is then repeated at regular intervals, you will continue reading and become oblivious to the sound.

A normal subject with closed eyes produces alpha waves on an EEG tracing. An auditory stimulation like a loud noise normally obliterates alpha waves for seven seconds or more. This is called "alpha blocking." However, in individuals who are not initiated in the art of meditation, the repeated sound stimulus will cease to have an impact on alpha blocking. In other words, there is a process of alpha habituation. Subjects become used to the novel stimulus once it is predictable. If the noise is repeated at fifteen-second intervals, studies find that, in normal subjects, there is virtually no alpha blocking by the fifth successive noise. Alpha habituation persists in normal subjects for as long as the noise continues at regular and frequent intervals.

In Zen masters, however, no habituation occurs. Their alpha blocking lasts two seconds with the first sound, two seconds with the fifth sound, and two seconds with the twentieth sound. This implies that Zen masters have a greater awareness of their environment as the result of meditative concentration. This capacity to stay present in the moment and the numinosity of each experience, rather than taking it for granted, is the fundamental property of the mindfulness practiced in Buddhism. Initiates in the art of mindfulness remain acutely aware of the present moment, with its mystery and awe, and never stop celebrating the gifts of the universe. A baby's smile, a colorful tree in autumn foliage, a full moon over a lake, a lover's smile, a friend's call—these things never cease to make their hearts skip a little beat! Most of us start taking these gifts for granted and even stop noticing them. When we look at a golden tree in late fall, we think of the impending winter rather than celebrating the golden autumn.

Gamma waves are a pattern of brain waves associated with perception and consciousness. They are produced when masses of neurons emit electrical signals at the rate of around forty times a second (40 Hz), but can often be seen between rates of 26 to 70 Hz. Researchers have recognized that higher-level cognitive activities occur when lower-frequency gamma waves suddenly double into the 40 Hz range (Lutz, 2004).

EEGs picked up a much greater than normal activation of fast-moving and unusually powerful gamma waves when Buddhist monks were the subjects of study. The movement of gamma waves through their brains was far better organized and coordinated. Meditation novices showed only a slight increase in gamma-wave activity while meditating, but some of the monks produced activity more powerful than any previously reported in a healthy person.

In meditation, long-term Buddhist practitioners self-induce sustained high-amplitude gamma-band oscillations and phase-synchrony patterns. Their EEG patterns differ from non-meditators, or "control" people, examined during these studies. In addition, the ratio of gamma-band activity (25–42 Hz) to slow oscillatory activity (4–13 Hz) is initially higher in the resting baseline before meditation for the practitioners than for the control group over medial front parietal electrodes. This difference increases sharply during meditation over most of the scalp electrodes and remains higher than the initial baseline in the post-meditation baseline. This data suggests that mental training involves temporal integrative mechanisms and may induce short-term and long-term neural changes.

It is not necessary to understand all the medical jargon here in order to appreciate the impact of these studies. Clearly, meditation has been shown to have identifiable and quantifiable physical effects, although it is too early to ascertain the clinical significance of these different EEG wave patterns in concentrated and mindful meditative states. Gamma-wave activity in mindfulness practitioners may, however, be reflective of higher states of consciousness more acutely attuned to the Healing Zone in the fourth dimension of consciousness, where the mind can be rebooted to a healthier attitude without the cognitive distortions that can turn into physical symptoms.

Conversely, once the mind is rebooted to a healthier and adaptive mode of functioning, this in turn may help reboot the body from a disease to a healthy threshold of functioning. This reflects the promise and the potential of the Healing Zone and may have significant impact on the mystery of mind/body medicine in the 21st century. To harvest the wonders of mind/body medicine, we must take baby steps into the fluid realm where mind and matter are in a quantum state of interchangeability. Meditation offers one avenue into this realm.

Different studies cite the virtues of both concentrated and mindful meditation. For the average person, however, these distinctions are academic. The best approach is to work with the method most comfortable for you. Most meditation techniques—including transcendental meditation, the jewel of the Indian tradition—blend contemplative and concentration methods. Transcendental meditation embraces concentration on a mantra and a passive attitude to receive the healing grace of the flow of the universe.

Healing through Meditation

- Find a quiet, solitary place in your house where you will not be disturbed for forty-five minutes.
- Sit in a comfortable chair or on the floor in a lotus position.
- Make sure you are not hungry, angry, lonely, or tired (HALT).
- Visualize that you are surrounded by a sphere of light. This sphere will protect you for the rest of your meditation exercise. Mentally calibrate this sphere of light to be larger or smaller until it feels right for you.
- Focus on your breath with intention. Always breathe in through your nose, then gently into your tummy, then gently out again. Stay focused on your breath.
- As you focus on your breath, note any distracting thoughts that come to mind. Gently put them outside of the sphere of light that protects you. Continue to focus on your breath.
- With each breath, feel a gradual wave of relaxation moving from the tips of your toes, up to your ankles, gradually up to your knees and hips, then up your spine all the way to the base of your skull and down both your shoulders, elbows, and wrists to the tips of your fingers. With each successive breath, feel the relaxation move from the base of your skull all the way to your crown and beyond.
- With each subsequent breath, focus your mind on your chosen repetitive word or mantra—"peace," "relax," "joy," etc.

- Maintain your body posture, surrounded by the sphere of protective light, and keep out all distracting thoughts. Focus on your breath with intention and reverence, gradually feeling the wave of relaxation all the way from the tips of your toes to the crown of your head. As you recite your personal mantra, continue to feel a sense of contemplative and deep relaxation.
- You will gradually feel a sense of inner peace and bliss as it descends on your mind and body. Experience that inner smile from your heart.
- Take five regular breaths. With each one, become more conscious of your body and your environment. First, feel your body, then the chair, then your body in the chair. Next, feel the chair's presence in the room, and then the presence of the room. After the fifth breath, gently open your eyes with a sense of joy and gratitude for the gift of breath, the gift of life, and the gift of the healing wisdom of the universe.
- Hold the intention that you will use these gifts to reach your personal best potentials, and that you will use these potentials in the service of family, community, and the God of your understanding. They will help you enter the Healing Zone.

Mindfulness

Mindfulness is the active awareness of your body, feelings, and thoughts, and your perception of objects, events, and individuals in your environment. It is the capacity to connect with the true nature of inner and outer reality without the distortions caused by the veil of maya through which you perceive others, the world, and yourself. This veil is created by distortions in your body, thoughts, and feelings, and in your perceptions of self, others, and the world. When you see the world through the veil of *maya,* your perceptions are transient and lead to suffering caused by your attempts to chase pleasure and avoid pain. Through mindfulness, you can realize that

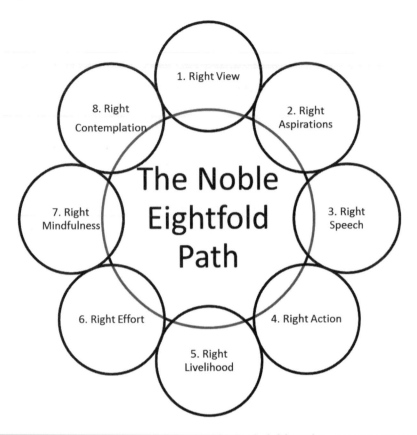

Figure 17. The Noble Eightfold Path.

your perceptions mire you in your ego and disconnect you from the transcendent reality of soul and Spirit (Gurnaratana, 2001).

Buddha provided a guide to mindfulness over 2,500 years ago. The Four Noble Truths of Buddhism include the truth of suffering, the truth of the cause of suffering, the truth of the end of suffering, and the truth of the path that leads to the end of suffering. Suffering is an aspect of the human condition; its cause is attachment to *samsara,* or life. The end of suffering, or *Nirvana,* entails a state of nonattachment or detachment. This state helps you attain *sunyata,* or the sacred void that makes room for kenosis—emptying the cup of your life and moving beyond superficial strivings. This in turn allows the divine, or Spirit, to emerge through a spiritually purposeful or dharmic life. The fourth Noble Truth charts the method for attaining the end of suffering. This is known to Buddhists as the Noble Eightfold Path (see figure 17). Once you attain this spiritual attitude through mindfulness, you experience the true nature of reality and the divine in the present moment. This connects you to the Healing Zone.

The steps on the Noble Eightfold Path are right view, right aspirations, right speech, right action, right livelihood, right effort, right mindfulness, and right contemplation. "Right" here implies following the guidance of your soul rather than doing the bidding of your ego and your complexes—the shadow, or lower, aspects of your personality.

Mindfulness involves engaging the present moment rather than remaining trapped in the past or being seduced by the future. By engaging the present moment, you begin to see both inner and outer aspects of reality more accurately, without the distortions of past experiences or future expectations. The present moment is the sacred realm that connects your history with your spiritual destiny.

Another important dimension of practicing mindfulness is that it moves you from experiencing ego to observing consciousness or inner witness. In so doing, you become an impartial but caring witness to your own experiences and body sensations, thoughts, and feelings, rather than becoming one with them. Through this, you learn that, when you are angry, you are not a bundle of anger. When you have neck pain, you are not the pain. If you have cancer, you are not the cancer; a part of your body has the cancer. This realization permits you to ally with the rest of your being as a witness to the whole picture rather than merging with the disease or dysfunctional part (see figure 18).

In practicing mindfulness, you realize that body sensations, thoughts, and feelings—and your perceptions of self, others, and the objects in your environment—are transient; they create impermanent states of pain or pleasure and are temporary constructs of

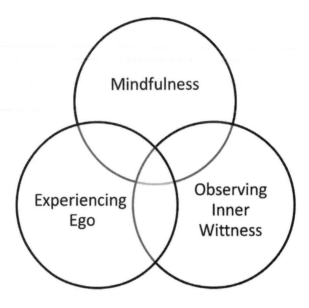

*Figure 18. The experiencing ego,
the inner witness, and mindfulness.*

your ego rather than stable attributes of your soul. You are free to release a body posture, a breathing irregularity, a thought distortion, or a faulty perception of others when you realize that these momentary experiences are not enduring, stable realities of your soul, but rather part of a world view you construct with your ego to pursue pleasure and avoid suffering. In mindfulness, you are free to observe life without getting caught in the ego distortions of maya.

As you observe inner reality more closely, you will find that happiness is not exclusively a quality brought about by a change in outer circumstances; it comes through centering yourself on your soul's guidance. Joy stems from loosening and releasing attachment to your hang-ups or complexes, which are the distorted lens through which you see the world. For example, if you have an inferiority complex, you assign tremendous power to others and relinquish your own authority. With a superiority complex or narcissistic personality, you inflate your own power and minimize the contribution of others in your life. Neither state is healthy or in tune with the larger reality of life.

Mindfulness does not have to be constrained to a formal meditation session. It is an activity that can be done at any time using pranayama, or breath management. Benedictine, Jain, Buddhist, Eastern Orthodox, and Hindu monks often practice a walking meditation and mindfulness. Any activity done mindfully is a form of meditation, and mindfulness is possible at practically any time.

In mindfulness, you focus on whatever activity you have undertaken with intention, deliberation, and total attention to every posture and movement. Instead of taking a "jitterbug" approach, you must slow down your activity by giving attention to every detail of your movements. If you are walking, feel mother earth supporting you with every step. If you are washing your car, feel the warmth of the water, the soft sponge, the sleek car, the cleansing soap, and the beautiful sunshine on your skin as you work. Be aware of your posture as you carry on the activity. Is your posture alert, flowing with the activity? Or is it rigid? Does the activity of your body cause you pain or pleasure? Remind yourself that whatever you are feeling in your body is transient and impermanent. Any attempt to avoid pain and seek pleasure is going to anchor your body in the illusion of maya. When you realize this transience, you can free your body and posture to align with the guidance of your soul and the intention of Spirit in the present moment. Your body then becomes an instrument of Spirit.

When you engage in body mindfulness, any activity becomes a yoga exercise connecting you with the flow of the healing energy of the universe. You can then experience the vein of joy and bliss beyond the discomfort of your body and the posture you are in. You can focus on the purpose your body has undertaken in the present rather than focus on your body itself.

When you undertake a mindfulness exercise—walking, sitting, or eating—focus on your breath. Is your breath regular or irregular? Slow or rapid? Rhythmic or chaotic? Nasal or oral? Are you breathing from your chest or from your abdomen? Is your breathing intentional or unconscious? Notice whether you can maintain focus on your breath, or if your mind jumps to other thoughts, images, feelings, or events.

The goal of breath mindfulness is to anchor your awareness to your breath. Your breathing should be slow and steady, systematic and nasal; breathe through your abdomen. Breathe without exertion, embracing all four steps of breathing—inhalation, abdominal retention of breath, exhalation, and external retention of breath—pacing each step to a count of three.

When your breath becomes unsteady, remind yourself that whatever distracts you is transient and will pass. If you are trying to perpetuate some pleasure or avoid pain, remind yourself that pain and pleasure are both impermanent and that chasing them only causes suffering. When you filter out these distractions, your breath will be steadied and will align with a deeper consciousness. It will become ready to join the flow of the universe and become a vehicle of the soul to do the work of Spirit. Breath mindfulness is one of the fastest and most expedient ways to center your monkey mind on a mindfulness track.

Often when dealing with patients in great pain or stress in psychotherapy sessions, I center myself by focusing on my own breath. This gives me a more helpful bodily and mental mindset in which to respond to the patient. I often invite patients to stay centered on their own breathing if they become anxious, panicky, dissociative, or emotionally fragmented when dealing with traumatic memories.

Inevitably, when practicing mindfulness, objects and individuals surround you. Some are experienced as pleasurable; others are painful. Some are desirable; some are disgusting. Usually, these perceptions, which are based on past experiences or future expectations, spin a veil of maya, or distortion, over your perceptions. The goal of mindfulness is to suspend judgment and anchor your perception in the present moment within a neutral frame—detached from pain or pleasure, desire or disgust. You must accept that, whatever your perception of an individual or event may be, it is transient and it too shall pass. Remind yourself that your perception is just a fleeting X-ray of a transient situation that is not the same as it was yesterday, and will not be the same tomorrow.

If an event, object, or individual calls for a response in the moment, respond in an authentic, sincere, detached manner to accomplish the task at hand—and then let go. If a friend drives you in his lovely sports car, enjoy the ride to your destination; do not get caught in admiration or envy of the friend and plan to get a similar or better car as soon as possible. With mindfulness, individuals and objects become vehicles of the soul, not the center of your desire.

This detached attitude helps you respond to the present moment so you can deal with outer reality, yet leaves you free to investigate the present in a deeper context and reflect on the more enduring or permanent aspects of the situation. This is the archetypal context of the present that shows how the present moment fits into the larger script of your life—your spiritual purpose, your dharma. It helps you put the moment in perspective and tunes you in to the dharmic, or spiritual, flow of your life, opening you to the energy flow of the universe. You can feel this in others who are guided by a sense of spiritual purpose. These individuals are old souls that have a certain unconscious aura about them. They attract us and make us feel good about the world and ourselves. Stay close to these people. In 12-step recovery programs, old-timers speak of this as "sticking with the winners."

Reflective, spiritually energized mindfulness opens up a vein of joy in your daily enterprise and lets you detach from the moment-to-moment pursuit of pleasure and avoidance of pain, encouraging you instead to dance to the deeper rhythm of life. Tuning in to your bliss body, soul, or Atman gives your consciousness a sharper focus. You can learn to manage the affairs of everyday life, while stepping back from them in favor of the deeper currents of your spiritual life. The experience is rejuvenating and health-restoring.

In practicing mindfulness, you experience a void in your ego consciousness from the absence of the ego's ceaseless chatter—the cause of your restlessness. We often confuse the serenity of the void with boredom. Only the initiated understand that the void is the sacred space that old souls try so hard to establish.

If you are bored of sitting still in mind and body, even for a short time, consider this: you are a passenger on mother-ship earth. The earth is spinning at about 1000 miles per hour at the equator and revolves at 66,000 miles per hour around the sun. The sun and the earth are moving at 48,300 miles per hour within the Milky Way and our galaxy is moving at 1.3 million miles per hour within the universe. If you can honor the void, you may experience the energy of the momentum of the universe flowing through you!

It takes tremendous courage and integrity to be true to your own nature. If you are practicing mindfulness and your mind strays to thoughts of making love to an attractive person, acknowledge your thought, your sensual nature, and guide it from lust to a soulful assessment of how you can transform your sensual nature from objectifying the person to relating to him or her as an individual soul—a living creature of God with a unique purpose in this lifetime. This does not negate your healthy attraction, but puts it into a larger spiritual context. You may find that this person attracts you beyond simple lust; perhaps grace and inner beauty beckons you. For men, this may prompt you to explore which part of your hidden grace and beauty the woman embodies and how you can live out this unlived part of your *anima,* or inner sacred feminine.

Mindfulness permits you to experience the moment in its full numinosity and engage the magic in the moment, whether it involves a pretty flower, a playful child, or a stranger's smile.

The experiencing ego is a function of the outer ego consciousness; the inner witness is a function of the soul. When these two do their dance, the resultant rhythm creates the music of mindfulness. I call this observing consciousness the "eagle consciousness," because it grants us an eagle's-eye view of ourselves. The sacred eagle is the totem bird for the observing consciousness.

Human consciousness is defined by the capacity to make choices. We can choose change or the status quo. One of the great human dilemmas involves balancing change with acceptance. Change must be guided by your soul and your spiritual path rather than by self-interest alone. However, you will always reach a crossroad where you will ask yourself: Should I struggle to change my situation or accept it? Mindfulness is a great guide at this crossroad. You should push for changes only when they are in harmony with your spiritual purpose. If this is not the case, you should accept your situation, trusting to God and the universe. This attitude moves you from maya and its karmic tangles to a dharmic, or spiritually engaged and purposeful, life. In the Hindu scripture the *Bhagwad Gita*, Lord Krishna counsels his protégé Arjuna on the yogic wisdom of engaging a spiritually purposeful, fully engaged life with detachment and mindfulness. "Work other than that done as a selfless service binds human beings," Krisha said. "Therefore, becoming free from selfish attachment to the fruits of work, do your duty efficiently as a service to Me."

The daily mindfulness exercise given below is designed to give you a soul's-eye view of yourself in contrast to the ego's view. In daily life—caught in maya, in the ego's chatter and concerns, and in the horizontal axis of your existence—you have little time for reflecting on the bigger picture. You devote little time to charting the sacred undercurrent of your existence, the meaning of your mundane life in the larger scheme of things. You are hard pressed to attend to your life in the context of family, neighborhood, city, country, and humanity.

When you are mindful of the eagle's view of yourself, you can realign your daily life with its eternal dimension and your momentary preoccupations with the eternal flow of life. Your finite existence can join with the infinite and absolute as best you understand it. Every moment, as mundane and trivial as it may seem, will then be infused with the purpose and the guidance of the sacred and its plan for you. When this bigger picture guides you, you feel focused, aligned, healthy, and whole. This feeling is the source of vitality and rejuvenation for your mind, body, and soul.

Elsewhere in this book, we have explored emerging research on the impact of mindfulness on the neurology of the brain. My speculation is that, in a gamma state of mindful meditative consciousness, the advanced practitioners observed in those studies were able to achieve a quantum state of consciousness in which mind, body, matter, and psyche were in a state of fluid interchangeability. Deep healing of the mind, body, and relationships can then transpire under the guidance of the soul. Gamma consciousness is also a matrix for the creation of new consciousness in the psyche, just as the gamma state of matter in the universe was the prerequisite for the creation of new matter and energy in the Big Bang.

Given sufficiently high frequency, gamma rays can transcend to a new state of being. When human brain-wave frequency crosses a certain threshold, the human psyche may create a new state of being for itself. The physical and psychological situations are mathematically equivalent. Once that frequency threshold is crossed, the system can spontaneously transform and transcend its state of being, arriving at a new state that is completely distinct from the old one. This transformation from sickness to healing is possible when we transcend the gamma state of consciousness through mindfulness, meditation, pranayama, and yoga. Perhaps this is the state of *samadhi,* or deep meditative mindfulness, spoken of by the rishis, the sadhus, and the yogis of ancient India, who aspired to transcend human suffering and experience the bliss body and soul consciousness in communion with the Primal Spirit—a place of fluid and healing continuity between mind, body, soul, and Spirit.

I believe that, in these mindfully mediated states of alpha and gamma consciousness, when a quantum state is activated, the reptilian, limbic, and neocortical brains become synchronized and bring all your ancient, ancestral, and archetypal wisdom and genetic heritage to bear on the process of repairing your illnesses. The experience transforms you into a state of health, healing, and wholeness.

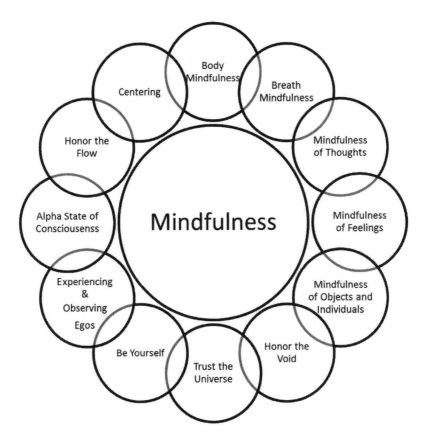

Figure 19. The practice of mindfulness.

All aspects of your being are aligned into an integrated whole and tuned in to the music of the universe. You become a vibrating string in the symphony of the cosmos. This deep state of consciousness can heal you and help you live out your fullest creative potential and spiritual purpose (see figure 19).

You will know that you are in this highly numinous state of consciousness when you experience a vein of joy in your being. When sustained for long enough, this joy permeates your mind, your body, and your soul with a sense of bliss that transcends individual consciousness and raises you into the collective consciousness.

You will feel one with the universe. Freud described this as an "oceanic feeling." Jung called it the *Unus Mundus*. Ancient Hindu sages and rishis called this deeply blissful state *samadhi*. This treasure is hard to attain. But with patience, practice, reverence, guidance, and wisdom, each of us has the potential to glimpse the sacred and numinous flow of the Healing Zone.

Practicing Mindfulness

When you do a mindfulness exercise in the context of aligning your thoughts, feelings, and actions to your soul, you are likely to harvest optimal health and spiritual dividends. Many researchers (Gurnaratana, 2001; Kabat-Zinn, 1990) have outlined excellent exercises for attending to the practice of mindfulness. Here is a simple one that I have found helpful in my own life and with some of my patients.

As you do this exercise, observe the objects and individuals in your immediate environment with respect, but with detachment. If your activity calls for you to engage them, do so in a brief, goal-directed manner. Do this exercise once daily with different activities, using some of the recommendations outlined above, but remembering to be flexible and to tailor them to your personality and circumstances.

- Begin in a quiet time and a secluded, comfortable place in your home. With experience, the practice of mindfulness can occur anywhere, at any time, and with any activity.
- Choose an activity during which you will practice mindfulness. This may be any number of things—going for a walk alone, eating a meal, organizing a desk or closet, cleaning the garage, mowing the lawn, doing dishes, or preparing a meal.
- Slow down the pace of the activity and do it with some degree of deliberation. Instead of rushing through the activity, do it intentionally, slowing your body and using systematic, methodical, intentional movements.

- While engaging in the activity, focus on your breath, slowing your breathing and using it as an anchor. Every few minutes, take five slow, deliberate breaths through your nose and into your tummy; be conscious of inhaling, holding in the air, and exhaling. Feel the prana, or breath energy, outside your nostrils. Throughout the rest of the exercise, continue to focus on your breathing as your anchor.

- Move in your mind from the activity itself to being the observer of the activity. Imagine that a part of you has become an eagle, flying overhead and observing your experience in relation to your surroundings, connections, or disconnections. The eagle now flies yet higher and observes you in an even wider relationship, eventually to the rest of the neighborhood. As the eagle continues to soar, it observes you in relationship to your city and country. At more advanced stages of mindfulness practice, you can imagine that your eagle is a satellite in orbit, observing you in a Google Earth view of yourself! By maintaining your eagle consciousness and detachment from the world, you can experience your pure soul consciousness.

- Once you are in this state of detached and pure eagle consciousness, begin noting your stream of thoughts, feelings, and experiences. Whatever they may be, receive them with love and put them in a safe vessel for attention later. Do not ignore them or get stuck in them, just receive them with love and acceptance, acknowledge them, and put them in this safe vessel as gifts from the Healing Zone. Do not think about them, manage them, or act on them. It must be as if you were watching a movie—just observing, not acting.

- Watch your thoughts and feelings as an eagle observer. Do they skip to the past or jump ahead into the future? Note your thoughts, but always place them into the safe vessel with love and acceptance.

- As you observe yourself from above with detached and pure consciousness and feel the sacred void in your mind, imagine

that you are alone in the presence of the sacred as you continue
your activity.

- Once you have completed your chosen task or activity, take
a few minutes to center yourself by sitting down in a chair or
on the ground. Fold your hands in reflection and feel the grace
of the sacred in your life. Thank the sacred eagle for giving
you a cosmic view of yourself from higher thresholds of consciousness. Thank the universe for the gifts of breath and life,
and the opportunity to serve humanity with every breath you
take. Remain anchored in your breath and return to regular consciousness, holding on to the rejuvenation and vitality you have
experienced.

Music and the Mind

Music can connect us with the Healing Zone. Immersion in soulful
music draws the strings of our hearts and souls. The music industry
knows this intuitively. Music touches us on the archetypal level
of the human psyche. It activates the limbic nervous system and
tunes in to the connection with the emotional body. For every mood
and occasion, we have a corresponding type of music—music for
joy and music for sadness, music for celebration and music for
loss, music for relaxation and music that activates mind, body, and
soul. The repertoire of Indian classical music includes ragas for the
morning and evening, for noon and night, for joy and sorrow, for
romance and regret, for exercise and relaxation, and for party and
prayer. Each is a bridge to the Healing Zone when used with intention, knowledge, wisdom, and reverence. In ancient India, the rishis
used *Gandharva,* or music therapy, to heal the mind, the body, and
the soul. Today, many young people use their favorite music for
quick access to healing and the vein of joy.

In neo-natal intensive-care units, music therapists use instruments that mimic heartbeats and womb sounds as well as their own

voices to comfort premature newborns and soothe them, to prepare them for feeding, and to help them sleep (Horne-Thompson, May 2008). Music therapy is also helpful for patients with anxiety, pain, and insomnia (Sarkamo, 2008). Besides promoting relaxation and reducing stress, music therapy has been shown to affect sleep patterns, improve stroke patients' memories, and decrease the amount of sedation needed for some patients.

In 2007, researchers conducted a randomized study in ten critically ill patients to identify mechanisms of music-induced relaxation using a selection of slow movements from Mozart piano sonatas (Conrad, et al., 2007). These sonatas were analyzed for compositional elements of relaxation. The researchers measured circulatory variables, electrical activity in the brain, serum levels of stress hormones and cytokines, requirements for sedative drugs, and levels of sedation before and after one-hour therapeutic sessions. They found that music significantly reduced the amount of drugs needed to achieve a comparable degree of sedation. Simultaneously, among those receiving music intervention, plasma concentrations of growth hormone increased, while interleukin-6 and epinephrine decreased. The reduction in these systemic stress-hormone levels was associated with significantly lower blood pressure and heart rate. Based on the effects of slow movements of Mozart's piano sonatas, they proposed a neurohumoral pathway by which music may exert its sedative action.

Another study examined the potential role of music in neurological rehabilitation (Sarkamo, et.al., 2008). This single-blind, randomized, and controlled trial was designed to determine whether everyday music listening can facilitate the recovery of cognitive function and mood after stroke. In the acute recovery phase, sixty patients with a left- or right-hemisphere middle-cerebral-artery stroke were randomly assigned to a music group, a language group, or a control group. During the following two months, the music and language groups listened daily to self-selected music or audio books, respectively, while the control group received no listening material. In addition, all patients received standard medical care and rehabilitation. All patients underwent an extensive neuropsychological assessment, which included a wide range of cognitive tests as well as mood and quality-of-life questionnaires. These were administered one week (baseline), three months, and six months after the stroke. Fifty-four patients completed the study. Results showed that recovery in the domains of verbal memory and focused attention occurred significantly faster in the music group than in the language and control groups. The music group also experienced less depression and confusion than the control group. These findings demonstrate for the first time that music listening during the early post-stroke stage can enhance cognitive recovery and prevent negative moods.

An Australian study examined the effectiveness of a single music-therapy session in reducing anxiety for terminally ill patients. Twenty-five participants with end-stage terminal disease were recruited. The experimental group received a single music-therapy intervention and the control group received a volunteer visit. The study found a significant reduction for the experimental group in anxiety, pain, and fatigue (Horne-Thompson, May 2008).

Again, it is not necessary to understand these medical protocols and results fully to understand that these studies indicate that music can have a significant impact on patients' physical symptoms and states. And today, the digital revolution has made the universe of music easily accessible to millions of individuals in a user-friendly form. The iPod and similar devices permit listeners to create playlists that invoke and kindle different moods to support wellness. I often recommend that my patients create playlists to support or activate different mood states. I have found that these playlists help activate or relax the sympathetic or parasympathetic nervous system pacemakers, depending on the task at hand. An emergency-room physician may have an activating, stimulating playlist to keep her going for hours dealing with trauma patients. The same surgeon may have another playlist on her iPod to help her relax once she is done with the day's work.

The iPod-based music-healing approach has been helpful for patients struggling with addictions, depression, anxiety, and somatic problems like irritable bowel syndrome or tension headaches. Whenever these individuals fall prey to cravings for drugs, alcohol, food, gambling, or pornography, a soothing, calming, relaxing playlist moves them from a stress response to a sober response to their thoughts, feelings, and behaviors.

With today's technology, it is easy to establish your iPod or CD player as your source of music for wellness. Consider putting iTunes or a similar program on your computer to create easily accessible playlists. Everyone has a favorite kind of music that helps them deal with different moods and situations. Create a playlist to deal with each of these moods: joy, sadness, anger, fear, shame, guilt. Whenever you feel one of these moods, play the list that, in your past experience, has reset your mood to one that is calm and joyful.

Create special playlists for play, exercise, reflection, contemplation, relaxation, etc.—one for increasing or toning down your energy level, one to wake you up in the morning, and one to help you gently fall asleep. Revise and update these playlists periodically and use them to reset your mood, and your anxiety and energy levels on a daily basis. Be sure to include some classical music along with the popular music. To activate your creative process, create a playlist that includes music in a foreign language, or from a different genre or culture. Have a special playlist to create a spiritual ambience. This can be very healing in time of crisis.

On the following pages are playlists created by my grandson, Signe Bedi, and a friend and trusted colleague, Dinshah Gagrat, that resonate with specific feelings.

Playlist by Signe Bedi

JOY:

- Orpheus in the Underworld, Galop Infernal—Offenbach
- Triumphant March—Verdi
- Blue Danube Waltz—Strauss

SADNESS:

- Hungarian Dance No. 5—Brahms (touching, occasionally energetic)
- Funeral March—Chopin
- Dies Irae—Mozart
- Clair de Lune—Debussy

ROMANCE:

- Rigoletto, La Donna e Mobile—Verdi
- Bourée in E minor—Bach (medieval in sound)
- Symphony No. 40 in G minor, Movement 1—Mozart

POWER AND ENERGY:

- Four Seasons, Winter—Vivaldi (stunning and, in cases, abrupt)
- Carmina Burana, O Fortuna—Orff
- Piano Sonata No. 11, Rondo Alla Turca (Turkish March)—Mozart
- Pictures at an Exhibition, Promenade—Mussorgsky (kingly)
- The Planets, Mars Bringer of War—Holst
- Symphony No. 9, Movement 1— DvoÝŠk (adagio, inspiring)
- Symphony No. 9, Movement 2—DvoÝŠk (allegro con fuoco, balanced)

Calming, soothing, comforting, centering:

- Bolero—Ravel (interesting)
- Cello Suite No. 1, Prelude—Bach (calming)
- Notturni, Liebestaum No. 3—Liszt

Spiritual ambiance, conveying a sense of the transcendent or divine:

- Symphony No. 7, Movement 2—Beethoven (allegretto, inspiring)
- Les trois gymnopédies—Satie (pensive, thought-provoking, centering)
- Cantata 147 (BWV), Jesu, Joy of Man's Desiring—Bach (calm)
- Pictures at an Exhibition, The Great Gate of Kiev— Mussorgsky

Playlist by Dinshah Gagrat

Joy:

- Ode to Joy—Beethoven
- Sonata for keyboard No. 8—Bach
- Symphony No. 5, Movement 4—Beethoven (allegro)
- Quintet in E-flat major for piano and winds—Beethoven

Sadness:

- Warsaw Concerto—Addinsell
- Piano Concerto No. 2, Movement 1—Rachmaninov (moderato)
- Piano Concerto No. 4 in G—Beethoven
- Rusalka, Act 1, O Silver Moon—DvoÝŠk
- Cello concerto in D, Meditation—Haydn
- Song without Words, Violin concerto in E Minor— Mendelssohn

ROMANCE:

- Water Music, Suite No. 1—Handel (The romantic connotation is that my wife was humming it the first time I met her. Subsequently, when my daughter got married, she walked down the aisle to this music)
- Rodelinda, Act 2—Handel
- Salut D'Amour—Elgar (written for his wife)
- Liebeslied—Liszt

POWER AND ENERGY:

- Symphony No. 5, Movement 1—Beethoven (allegro con brio)
- Concerto for cello and orchestra in E Minor—Elgar
- Cello Concerto No.1 in C, Movement 3—Haydn (allegro molto)
- Cesare in Egitto, Va tacito e nascosto—Handel
- Barber of Seveille, Dunque io son—Rossini
- Variations on a Rococo Theme—Tchaikovsky
- Violin Concerto in D— Tchaikovsky

SOOTHING:

- Goldberg Variations—Bach
- Violin Concerto in E minor—Mendelssohn
- Quintets for Piano and Winds—Mozart (largo, allegro, larghetto)
- Clarinet Quintet in A— Mozart
- Piano Sonata No. 13 in A—Schubert (allegro moderato)
- Cello Concerto No. 2 in D—Hob
- Violin Concerto in E minor, Movement 2—Mendelssohn (andante)

Mandalas and Brain-Wave Training

In therapy, I have found that the soul offers patients prescriptions in the form of healing images if they draw a mandala or make a collage of a resolution to a problem. When they hold this image and its accompanying emotions in consciousness, a new reality starts to emerge in their lives. It is as if the image rewires the brain, which lays out new consciousness. In this new consciousness, patients see possibilities and choices that did not exist in their old consciousness. Engaging this new consciousness, with its corresponding menu of choices, opens up a wider repertoire of behaviors. More adaptive behaviors create a new reality, fulfilling and nurturing the mind, body, and soul. By coupling a new image with an old problem, they engage the Healing Zone and are able to break out of the old paradigm into auspicious new beginnings. This takes courage and sacrifice.

Jenny is a good example of how mandalas can function as healing images. Jenny was a workaholic health professional who sought treatment and therapy for depression and loneliness. She lived a monastic life and was over-involved in work as a diversion and defense against fear of engagement in the other sectors of her life. My usual counsel to work on life/work balance bore no major dividends. She understood my point intellectually, but something kept blocking her attempts to engage other sectors of her life. Love, relationships, and play were in the blind spot of her existence. Since Jenny was interested in drawing and art, I invited her to make a collage of her lonely life and her image of healing this void. The following week, she brought a beautiful collage—a mandala image of a tea party with a few close friends. In real life, she did not have any close friends, but the visual image became a focus of our therapy.

I counseled Jenny to keep this mandala in her consciousness and to see what happened. Over the next few weeks, she began a friendship with a colleague at work and they started meeting during their tea breaks at the hospital. This synchrony between the tea-party mandala and real life gained momentum. She started to socialize more and get out of her lonely shell. A few weeks later, she dreamed of her high school class reunion. In this dream, she encountered James, her old boyfriend. She felt betrayed, deeply wounded, and abandoned when James started to date her best friend. This exacerbated the abandonment she had felt as a child by her workaholic father. Jenny became fearful of relationships and those early wounds became obstacles to any relationship in later life. Yet a big part of her was ready to break out of this shell. Her depression became a call to reset this dynamic. When she engaged the void, her soul blessed her with the image of a tea party, which became a paradigm for her to climb out of her black hole and back into life. Jenny was ready to join the tea party of life.

Jung was convinced of the healing power of mandala images. Based on his theory, researchers Olga Grechko and Vladimir Gontar proposed that visual stimuli in the form of mandalas can provide a therapeutic effect through neurofeedback training, a form of biofeedback that attempts to train EEG brain-wave patterns (Grechko, 2009). Their biofeedback system applies a mathematical model to transform an online recording of EEG signals and a simulated time-series EEG into a computer-generated series of mandala images reflecting the subject's mental state. They demonstrated what the ancients suspected—that brain activity can be represented as a mandala.

Neurofeedback training is a fascinating area with considerable potential to help us engage the Healing Zone. In an article in the *Scientific American Mind*, Ulrich Kraft reviews the history and present status of neurofeedback training in treating attention deficit, epilepsy, and depression, along with boosting concentration and creativity in pilots and musicians (Kraft, 2006). In neurofeedback, an EEG is used to give ongoing feedback via a computer to help bring brain waves into a desirable range using positive reinforcement. Reinforcing the low beta frequencies in the sensory-motor cortex of the brain reduces proneness to seizure or epilepsy. Sufferers of attention-deficit hyperactivity disorder with a low level of beta waves can also be helped by increasing their beta frequency through neurofeedback training. Richard Davidson's research found that depressed patients have a higher distribution of alpha activity in the anterior part of the right frontal lobe and diminished alpha activity in the anterior part of the left frontal lobe (Davidson, 1995). Following this research, psychologists J. Peter Rosenfeld, Elsa Baehr, and Rufus Baehr used neurofeedback training to boost the alpha activity on the left frontal lobe with positive initial results (Baehr, et al, 1999).

Neurofeedback promises to shed the light of medical science on many ancient paths into the Healing Zone and has yielded some amazing successes for patients previously responding poorly to psychotherapy and psychotropic medications. Along with reduction in symptoms and a seemingly biological fix came an unexpected change in personality and philosophical outlook on life and others.

In Jung's (1960) essay on psychic energy, he repeatedly acknowledged the limitations of the science of his time, especially the lack of ways to quantify the energy of the mind. Without the means to use the objectivity of scientific experimentation, he had to resort to his empirical observations in his clinical setting. When I revisited Jung's *Collected Works*, I learned that he abandoned his work with the "psychoganvinator" and "pneumograph," very rudimentary biofeedback instruments he used with word-association tests to observe physiological responses better. I wonder if today he might return to the quantitative approach because of the sophisticated electronic EEG amplifiers and amazing computer software now available. I believe Jung's curiosity surely would have led him to revisit a scientific approach. We may finally have the means to quantify the energy of the psyche and to study the neurological patterns parallel to the complexes scientifically. What follows is a humble first attempt to go beyond the alchemy of Jungian psychology toward a renaissance of the archetypal with modern neuropsychophysiology, the chemical/electric mix of the mind (Jung, 1973).

In his clinical work with neurofeedback, Dr. David Drapes began to see a parallel between controlling brain waves and controlling complexes. He observed that changes in brain-wave patterns caused changes in mental images and metaphors. Could there be a connection to psychic energy? Could archetypes be playing a role? A quick return to an old Jolande Jacobi classic surprised him with a diagram of an "energic" wave. According to Jacobi: "The nuclear element has a constellating power corresponding to its energic value…it is a kind of 'neuralgic point,' a centre of functional disturbance, which becomes virulent…From an active, conscious state the individual falls into a passive 'seizure'" (Jacobi, 1951).

One of the most medically successful uses of neurofeedback is treatment for the control of epilepsy. The type of EEG training Drapes selected for his inquiry was a conservative protocol backed by over forty years of experimental and clinical research and used by the astronauts—sensory motor rhythm (SMR). This is the same treatment protocol used to help control epilepsy. This led Drapes to ask a key question: If seizures—thunderstorms of the mind—can be contained, perhaps complexes and their emotion-toned energy can also be controlled or guided in a positive direction.

SMR procedure entails the placement of a sensitive electrode on the top center of the head and on the earlobes. The subject then observes his/her brain waves on a computer screen in real time. Pre-programmed software separates the brain-wave frequencies for training. The training involves operant conditioning of the pre-selected protocol. For SMR training, low theta waves (4–8 Hz) and high beta waves are inhibited, while low beta waves (12–15 Hz) are reinforced. The goal is to influence the thalamus in the lower, mid, unconscious, and automatic part of the brain.

The thalamus is the relay station of brain-wave activity. It is also metaphorically considered the "conductor" of the symphony of the brain. Theoretically, the thalamus is active in pattern recognition and, like Pavlov's dog, can be conditioned. With neurological feedback, the thalamus can be trained to relay/conduct specified brain-wave patterns. It has been shown experimentally that, in most cases, the training is retained—much as we maintain our ability to ride a bike or to swim once our bodies are conditioned to those activities.

The analogy of the symphony in the brain can also help us understand how EEG brain-wave training and complexes may be related. If we see role of the conductor as that of the ego, and if the ego is not a strong or competent conductor, the orchestra can easily lose its rhythm. Neurologically, it can become "dysregulated." When this happens, the mind exhibits psychological and/or physiological symptoms. Anxiety, ADHD, depression, and a hyperactive autonomic nervous system are but a few examples.

Returning to our analogy, if we see the role of the conductor is weak or not present, the orchestra can be taken over by one of the sections, which then imposes its will and rhythm on the entire ensemble—in this case, the mind. In our analogy, the section that takes over is like the complex that takes over and exerts its pattern over the psyche. The brain is then at the mercy of the complex—the dysregulated brain-wave pattern. This pattern will continue until the conductor, the ego, retakes control or the brain-wave pattern is trained/conditioned through neurofeedback.

Another fitting analogy, a favorite of Jung's, may be that the sections of the orchestra—parts of the brain—represent the gods or the archetypes. When the gods are in dysrythym, they become symptomatic. They are our dysregulated brain-wave patterns. All the gods must be honored in a symphonic way that requires an experienced, healthy, and balanced conducting ego. Without a strong ego, we are vulnerable to the winds of past trauma, the whims of our fears, and the revenge of the gods for not being honored equally.

Brain-wave training involves one to two sessions per week.

The actual neurofeedback lasts about thirty minutes. The length of neurofeedback treatment varies from twelve to forty sessions. The real-time display allows patients to observe changes in their own brain-wave patterns. Their awareness of the change and their ability to alter the pattern is possible due to the neuroplasticity of the brain. The brain has the ability to control and to grow itself, if it has the appropriate type of feedback. Patients not only see their brain waves; they also watch software-created patterns in the form of computer images and games. The games are designed to reinforce desirable patterns by positive visual and auditory feedback. They are like symbols; the challenges of the games are analogous to the path and toils of the Hero. The session is a transformative mini-exercise in the growth of the psyche, as well as in the growth of brain cells and interconnections.

Examples like Jung's case studies add an empirical and subjective element to treatment for patients from an objective view. The objectivity of hard science adds a perspective that can turn life's labyrinthine patterns into a mandala—a map. When the heat of the human story of struggle is combined with the cold dispassion of hard technology, a transforming container is constructed in which a new alloy can be created.

As important as the number of brain-wave changes are, however, the goal of neurofeedback is always a positive change in the patient's attitude and behavior. The numbers can give guidance when the patient is lost in the darkness of life or the dysrythm of synaptic fog. When a complex takes over, science now gives us a tool on which patients can focus to see an electrical pattern of the problem. They can then exert some control over the cognitive component of the complex.

Joe, a man in his mid-sixties, requested neurofeedback to help control his epilepsy. After a number of EEG training sessions, he was not only pleased with the positive results in controlling the seizures, but also pleasantly surprised that his past negative view of life had changed. He noted that he had become more loving toward his wife and now wanted to reunite with his son, from whom he had been estranged for many years. Joe stated that he believed that the Type-A behavior he had exhibited for much of his adult life had evolved into Type-B patterns in which he felt more relaxed, less emotionally reactive, and able to disassociate with ease from past patterns. He was no longer enslaved by episodic irritability brought on by his impatience with others' "stupid and slow" behavior. Joe marveled at his changed energy level, his new-found love of life, and his love of others. He was delighted with the loss of his past hypercritical habits.

Creating Your Personal Mandala

In neurofeedback, an EEG is used to give ongoing feedback via a computer to help bring brain waves into a desirable range using positive reinforcement. You can work toward the same goals yourself, without the aid of technology, using this mandala exercise.

- Identify the life situation or problem to which you want to attend.
- Make a collage that represents your response to this problem.
- Keep this collage in mind when you are dealing with the problem.
- Note the thoughts, feelings, sensations, and possibilities that this image stimulates in you.
- Note the synchronistic events that emerge as you keep this collage in your consciousness.
- Note any dreams that arise that relate to this collage. For example, if your problem is loneliness and difficulty in establishing or sustaining a relationship, note if you dream about your ex-boyfriend who betrayed you and started dating your best friend.
- Note how these early wounds get in your way now. Do you shun relationship opportunities for fear of betrayal?

- Take back the power from the wound and empower yourself to take charge of your life and open yourself to new possibilities after due discernment.
- Practice this new paradigm to reinforce it.

Yantras

Yantra, a Sanskrit word, derives from the root *yam,* meaning "to sustain or hold." In metaphysical terms, a yantra is visualized as a receptacle of the spiritual essence of your latent code. A yantra can take the form of an instrument, apparatus, talisman, or mystical diagram whose purpose is to activate the Healing Zone.

The sacred geometry of a yantra works by balancing the dimensions of the personality—including mind, body, soul, and your connection with Spirit. A yantra realigns the five basic elements of nature (earth, water, fire, air, and sky) in the body and psyche by recitation of certain mantras. The Jungian alchemical tradition has explored this balance of elements in the personality in great detail. Meditation on a yantra helps you balance your personality under the archetypal guidance that is relevant to your life situation. It may, for instance, balance the excessive fiery nature of your personality with the cooling water of a less-explored aspect of yourself.

Every yantra is based on a balance of masculine and feminine. Yantras help rebalance your masculine and feminine energies symbolically, maintaining them in the proportion necessary to respond to your present needs. It is important to note here that the concept of masculine and feminine in analytical psychology is different than in the lay use of these terms. These are not gender-based attributes; both genders have so-called masculine and feminine attributes in varying proportions unique to each individual. Jung tried to get around any gender bias by coining the terms *anima* for the feminine psyche and *animus* for the masculine. For our purposes, masculine energy involves a sense of initiative and enterprise in both men and women; feminine energy refers to a sense of value and feeling for both sexes. For instance, to deal with a professional challenge, you may need to use masculine initiative as well as to make feminine value judgments.

A yantra symbolically represents the human body and psyche. Most are circles enclosed in a square outer form with four gates. The square represents the ego consciousness, while the circle represents the unconscious. Whenever something unconscious becomes conscious, it is symbolized by a circle, or a round shape, becoming a square or a cube. The square outer layer of a yantra represents the act of entering the circle, or the unconscious, via consciousness. Dreams, on the other hand, involve the unconscious entering into consciousness. The goal is to establish a bridge between the square and the circle, between the conscious and the unconscious, between the ego and the Healing Zone. The eternal dance of squaring the circle and circling the square is essential for your transition from illness to wellness.

Each archetype is activated by a specific yantra, which acts like a password that opens up the immense energies and possibilities inherent in the archetype (see figures 20–23). By regularly meditating on a specific yantra, you can tune in to the corresponding archetype to focus its healing energies in your psyche and foster personal growth.

The circle represents the unconscious aspects of your personality that must be squared, or made conscious. Consciousness, represented by the square, has four doors that open to four functions, four elements, and four seasons to comprehend the outer world. This permits the lotus within (the soul) to blossom into wholeness with eight petals. At the heart of the unceasing dance between square and circle is a process of cooperation, mutuality, and engagement between your consciousness and your unconscious to unfold your immense potential for wellness. Integrating the opposite tendencies in your psyche involves fusing your masculine and feminine sides, your ego with its shadow, your thinking with feeling, your intuition with attention to details, your consciousness with your unconscious, your personal fulfillment with community welfare, your soul with Spirit, your human enterprise with the wisdom of the universe.

When you meditate on a yantra, you try to project different aspects of your personality onto the symbols of the yantra. Where are the earth, water, fire, and air aspects of your nature located in your present personality? What are the representations of your masculine and feminine potentials in the circle? Do you have a feeling for your *bindu* (the point that represents the soul) in the mandala circle? Does the yantra align your *bindu* with the energies and intentions of the universe? Does your present life situation feel black, white, green, golden, or red?

Saraswati Yantra

The Saraswati yantra helps you focus the energy of the archetype for the goddess Saraswati, the patron of artists and academics, in your personal consciousness. The goddess guides not only teachers, students, and artists, but also anyone who undertakes a new course of study or education. The Saraswati yantra has two triangles at its core, symbolizing the perfect union of masculine and feminine energy (see figure 20). In beginning a new course of education, you must honor the masculine and feminine perspectives equally to acquire the optimal attitude to the subject being studied. You need feminine guidance to discern what is of value and masculine initiative to pursue it rigorously.

Eight petals surround the Saraswati yantra; the number eight is a symbol of infinity. The latent code of Saraswati opens up the realms of knowledge and infinite possibilities. To really experience your soul, you must prepare your consciousness with attention to academics and an artistic eye for life. Knowledge imparted by the code of Saraswati is a source of power, for knowledge is power. It is only with respect for sacred words and speech that you can rekindle

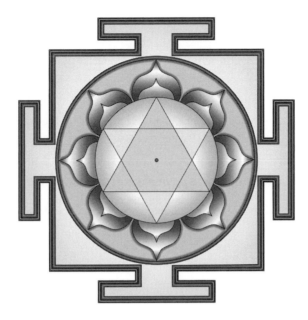

Figure 20. Saraswati yantra.
See also Plate 2, color insert following page 160.

your relationship with Spirit and the universe and regenerate your personal consciousness in accord with your spiritual roots.

The mantra for Saraswati's latent code is *Om Sri Vidya Dayeni Saraswatiye Namaha*, which means: "O great Universe, my salutations to goddess Saraswati. May she impart to me the necessary knowledge and wisdom to fulfill my spiritual responsibilities in this lifetime."

Sri Yantra

By invoking the archetype of Laxmi, goddess of fortune and beauty, the Sri yantra guides you, not only to material prosperity, but also to inner peace and the spiritual realignment of your life in accord with the program of the universe. The Sri yantra aligns the various opposing aspects of your psyche—masculine and feminine, solar

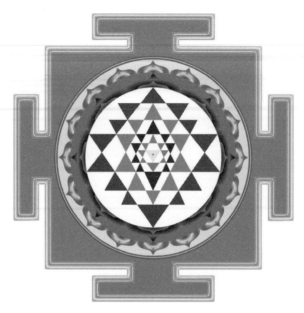

Figure 21. Sri yantra.
See also Plate 3, color insert following page 160.

and lunar, fire and water, earth and sky—to a central point or bindu that represents the consciousness of your soul. The surrounding geometries represent the unfolding of the creative possibilities in the psyche when you are centered in the bindu or soul. These infinite creative possibilities are inspired by the latent code of Laxmi.

The Sri yantra is composed of two sets of triangles (see figure 21). One set includes four male triangles denoting the four aspects of evolved or limited consciousness. The other set includes five female triangles denoting the five vital functions, the five senses of knowledge, the five senses of action, and the five subtle and five physical forms of matter.

These two sets of triangles are superimposed to show the union of the masculine and feminine aspects of your nature. When united, they make the figure within the eight lotus petals of the yantra. Four gates or doors, called *bhupura*, surround these triangles, representing the gates of the consciousness to the deeper mysteries beyond.

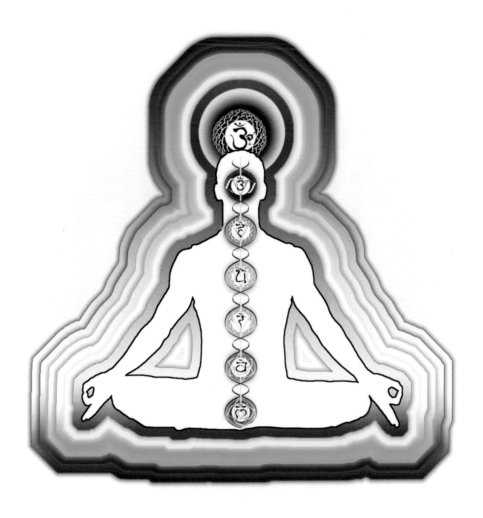

Plate 1: The eight preparatory steps on the path to yoga.

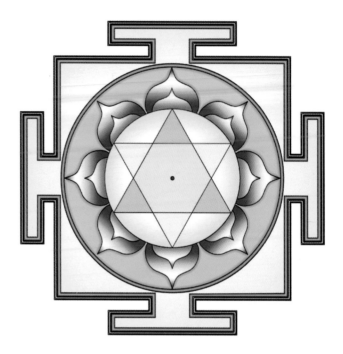

Plate 2: Saraswati yantra

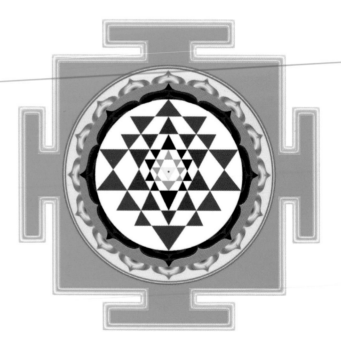

Plate 3: Sri yantra

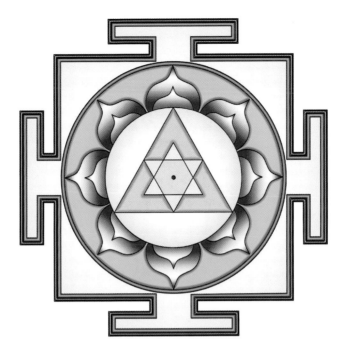

Plate 4: Ganesha yantra

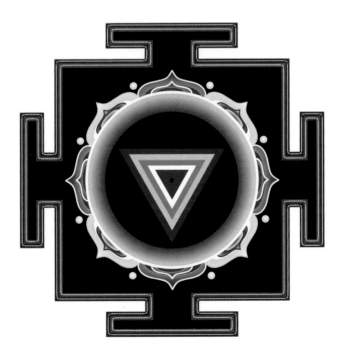

Plate 5: Kālī yantra

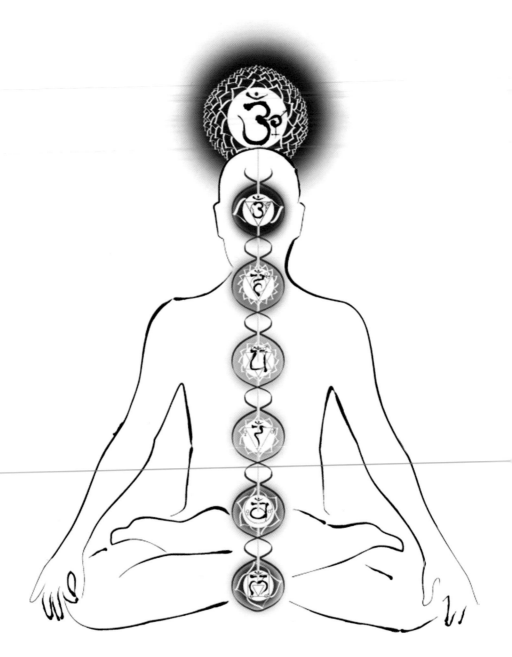

Plate 6: The path of Kundalini energy

The Sri yantra also has nine *cakras,* or compartments, formed by the intersection of the triangles.

The Sri yantra's red central point, or bindu, is the point of bliss, standing for divinity and the Mother as the source from whence everything represented in this diagram proceeds. Red is the active color of passion for what is valuable about life and the color of the latent code of evolving Laxmi consciousness.

The object of worshipping this yantra is to attain unity with its latent code. You can transform the yantra in your consciousness from a material object of lines and curves into a mental state of union with the universe and its divine essence. You thus become one with the Sri yantra, and realize its healing potential.

The mantra for the Sri yantra is *Om Shri Mahalaxmiye Namah,* which means: "Salutations to the Great Goddess Laxmi."

Ganesha Yantra

The Ganesha yantra illustrates the dance of the circle and the square, with the circle representing the unconscious aspects of the psyche that are squared or made conscious. This allows your consciousness to harvest the hidden treasures of the unconscious to fulfill your tasks. The square has four doors that open to your four functions, four elements, four seasons, and the wholeness of consciousness. This permits the lotus within (the soul) to blossom into the wholeness represented by the eight petals. Masculine and feminine energies are thus integrated into a hermaphrodite soul.

At the core of the Ganesha yantra stands an upright masculine triangle and the reverse feminine triangle (see figure 22). This signifies the balance necessary for making positive beginnings. Even so, both triangles are enclosed in another upright masculine triangle. This signifies the need for masculine initiative to make a new beginning and calls for a dynamic masculine enterprise. You must be ready to sacrifice old attitudes, as in the myth of Ganesha, to make room for a new outlook on life. However, once the dynamic

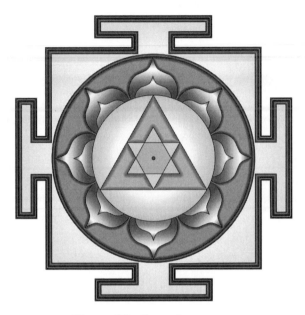

Figure 22. Ganesha yantra.
See also Plate 4, color insert following page 160.

masculine energy is activated, you must make room for the balanced representation of masculine and feminine perspectives if these energies are to have an enduring and beneficial effect.

The eight petals of the Ganesha yantra symbolize infinity, or the wholeness of the psyche. The color rose symbolizes the soul, as well as the planet Mars, representing empowerment of the soul. The color red also symbolizes the sacrifice of Ganesha, the process of atonement for the sins of your ancestors, and the regeneration of your higher psychic potential.

The mantra for the Ganesha yantra is *Om Ganeshaye Namah,* which means: "Salutations to Ganesha."

Kālī Yantra

Kālī represents the disintegrative force in nature, as displayed in the passage of time and an increase in entropy. Kālī is symbolized in the yantra as black (see figure 23). The downward-pointing tri-

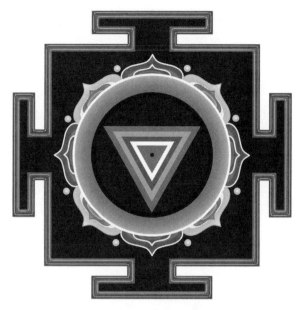

Figure 23. Kālī yantra.
See also Plate 5, color insert following page 160.

angle is an ancient symbol of the primal female, the origin of all things—the pubic triangle of the Great Goddess.

The eight-petal lotus is the eight-fold Prkriti, or nature, consisting of earth, water, fire, air, ether, *manas* (mind), *buddhi* (intellect), and *ahamkara* (ego). The five triangles are the five *jnanendriyas* (*jnana* means "knowledge"; *indriyas* means "the senses"), the five *karmendriyas* (motor organs), and the five pranas (breathing activities). The bindu at the center is the symbol of the balanced soul. The five triangles also represent the sacred marriage of the feminine and masculine aspects of your psychological potential. They correlate with a host of sacred symbols, including the Seal of King Solomon, the five letters in the name of Jesus and his five wounds, as well as the sacred Pentagram. All five triangles are essentially feminine. They point downward, symbolizing the essence of the Kālī yantra as compensating for an excessive masculine drive in the personality.

The Kālī yantra is invoked when you are dealing with a major life crisis or trauma. It activates the latent code of Kālī for the purpose of survival and mastery of an overwhelming situation. Invoke Kālī when your ego consciousness runs into a dead-end and you feel that there is no way out. When your ego surrenders to the universe, the code of Kālī is activated to guide your path through the darkness into light. The hidden potentials of your personality rise when ego and pride step out of the way. The way of Kālī overcomes your ego attitude to your adversities, enabling you to see a reflection of yourself in the mirror of your adversaries.

The mantra to guide your consciousness through the Kālī yantra meditation is *Om Kareeng Kalekaye Namah,* which means: "Salutations to Goddess Kālī."

Creatinge Your Personal Yantra

Creating a personal yantra gives you a scan of the state of your own psyche in the present moment and opens up the possibility of correcting any energy imbalances in your personality.

• Focus on a life problem, a relationship tangle, a medical or psychiatric problem, a crisis, a trauma, or a major life decision that lies ahead of you. Write it down and keep it in your consciousness as you construct your yantra.

• Draw a square to represent your conscious assessment of the situation or problem. Each side of the square represents one aspect of your problem.

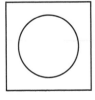

• Insert a circle in the square to represent your fears and concerns about the problem—your unconscious response to the conscious problem.

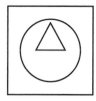 • Insert an upward-facing triangle to represent your active efforts to attend to this problem. This represents your masculine response. If you have been very active, you may insert more than one upward-facing triangle.

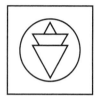 • Insert a downward-facing triangle to represent how passive you have been in dealing with this problem. If you have been more passive than active, you may insert more downward-facing triangles. (In the example to the left, you are twice as passive as you are active.)

- Add a point, or bindu, to represent your center in the yantra.
- Decide whether the situation calls for a more active response or a more passive, wait-and-see response. If the ratio of masculine to feminine triangles is what it needs to be, that's fine. If not, decide whether the situation calls for more activity or passivity.
- Decide how you plan to be consciously more active or passive. This will represent your gates, or escape, out of your dilemma. Now *do it!*

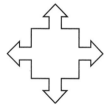 • Color this square with blue, black, white, yellow, or red. Blue represents openness to the universe for guidance on your next move; black represents the uncertainty or mess you may experience in your present predicament. White symbolizes mental clarity about your dilemma; yellow invokes spiritual guidance; red is the color of embodiment, action, and determination to take the plunge into the river of life to deal with your issues. Choose the color that resonates with your level of engagement with your present situation.

Kundalini Balancing

Kundalini yoga is one of the most sophisticated systems for accessing the Healing Zone and rejuvenating your mind, body, and soul in accord with your spiritual purpose. Kundalini focuses on the coiled serpent at the base of the spinal column at the root of the body, calling it to ascend through the seven chakras—the synapses of mind, body, and soul—to reach the seventh (or crown) chakra, the place of your highest potential and connection to Spirit or the flow of the universe (see figure 24).

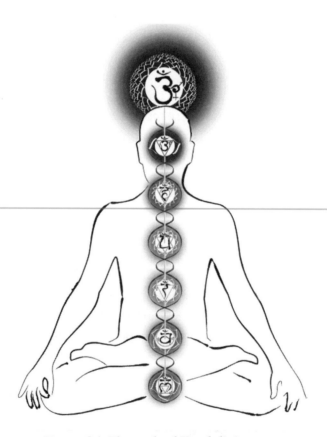

Figure 24. The path of Kundalini energy.
See also Plate 6, color insert following page 160.

At each of these seven synapses or junctions, you can balance your masculine and feminine energies and sort out your relationship and mind/body imbalances with the help of a specific archetypal gatekeeper (see Tables 1 and 2). When you are balanced in the root, or first, chakra, you are ready to move to the second, and so on up the ladder until you mature and reach the seventh. Being stuck at any of these seven synapses can cause medical or psychiatric symptoms like relationship problems and psychological developmental blocks. Carl Jung was fascinated by Kundalini yoga and did a series of seminars on it (Jung, 1996). Jungian analysts Vasavada and Spiegelman have done a detailed Jungian treatise on this subject (Spiegelman and Vasvada, 1987).

Table 1. Kundalini Archetypal Balancing			
Kundalini Synapse	Archetypal Guide	Archetypal Split	Developmental Balance
root chakra	Mother	abandonment/ engulfment	basic trust
second chakra	Father	control/ shame, doubt	autonomy, generativity, creativity
third chakra	Warrior	control/initiative; industry/ inferiority	initiative, enterprise, mastery
fourth chakra	Lover	intimacy/isolation	intimacy, mutuality
fifth chakra	Trickster	ego identity/ ego confusion	ego identity, finding your own voice
sixth chakra	Leader	generativity/ stagnation	leadership
seventh chakra	Guru/ Teacher/ Mentor	ego integrity/ despair	spiritual attitude, capacity to mentor younger generations

Table 2. Kundalini Relationship Balancing				
Kundalini Synapse	Archetypal Guide	Relationship Tangles	Relationship Balance	Developmental Balance
root chakra	Mother	aggressor/ victim	self-mothering	basic trust
second chakra	Father	exploiter/ martyr	self-parenting	autonomy, generativity, creativity
third chakra	Warrior	master/slave	partner	initiative, enterprise, mastery
fourth chakra	Lover	caretaker/ dependent	mutuality	intimacy, mutuality
fifth chakra	Trickster	intimidator/ silent	communicator, finding your own voice	ego identity, finding your own voice
sixth chakra	Leader	leader/ follower	participator	leadership
seventh chakra	Guru/ Teacher/ Mentor	narcissistic/ autistic	teacher, mentor, guru, guide	ego integrity, capacity to mentor younger generations

Energy moves through the chakras in three channels called *nadis*. Each nadi is a motor system and is automatic in the sense that most of its functions are carried out below the threshold of consciousness.

The sympathetic nervous system corresponds to the *pingala nadi*. This is the "hot" system that prepares the body for the fight-or-flight response. In general, it excites the heart and blood vessels, increasing blood pressure, slowing the gastro-intestinal system, and increasing the metabolism of every cell in the body. Pingala is the carrier of intellectual/mental energy. It makes the physical body more dynamic and more efficient, and provides increased vitality and "male" power. Pingala has a purifying effect, but its cleansing is like fire.

The *ida nadi* corresponds to the parasympathetic system—the "cool" system responsible for calming, soothing, and renewing. It has a more discriminative, organ-specific response pattern than the sympathetic nervous system. In general, it calms the heart, lowers blood pressure, enhances the gastro-intestinal system, and is responsible for sexual stimulation and functioning. The ida nadi is the channel of physical/emotional energy. It is "feminine" in nature, the storehouse of life-producing, maternal energy. Ida nourishes and purifies, but its purification is gentle.

When Kundalini energy is concentrated in one or the other of these nadis, the result is an energy imbalance correlating to Type-A or Type-B personalities. When energy moves primarily in the "hot" pingala nadi, the result is a Type-A personality who is always on the go. Type-A people are characterized as competitive and hard-driving, impatient and verbally aggressive, and prone to anger and hostility. These characteristics appear to be associated with increased risk of cardiovascular disease. From a Kundalini point of view, the pingala nadi is overly energized in these individuals.

On the other hand, when Kundalini moves primarily in the "cool" ida nadi, individuals show Type-B characteristics. Type-B personalities tend to be cooperative, easy-going, and patient, and have a generally mellow temperament. The desirable condition is for neither nadi to dominate, but rather for energies to flow naturally and in balance through the third nadi, the central channel called the *sushumna*.

This balance can be achieved in two ways. You can consciously and intentionally strengthen the flow in one nadi and decrease it in the other; or you can experience a transformation so that the energy flows in the central sushumna nadi. Maintaining the tension between pingala and ida demands consciousness and self-discipline. Eventually, the tension may resolve when the energy begins to flow through the sushumna. In a Type-A person, this means a decrease in compulsive self-assertion, replaced by greater flexibility to choose how to address issues and situations. A Type-B person may still be laid-back and easy-going, but may become more assertive when situations call for an energetic response.

The nadis are linked with the chakras, which are the subtle energy centers of interchange between the physical, emotional, psychological, mental, and spiritual dimensions. Medical and psychological symptoms often indicate that one or more chakras are over- or under-energized, and that you are stuck in either the ida or pingala nadi in one or more chakra.

When you live predominantly in either the hot or cool nadi, the unlived potential of the under-energized nadi automatically finds expression in illness or by projecting your past experience onto a significant person in your present life—a spouse, parent, employer, friend, or adversary.

The seven Kundalini chakras are subtle energy points where the somatic, psychic, and spiritual dimensions of your being intersect. Each person has a dominant chakra where personal or individual dharma resides. The other six chakras are auxiliary chakras that inform, assist, and complete the optimal achievement of your dharma, which is situated in your dominant chakra. No one chakra is superior or inferior to the others. They mediate different aspects of energy and you must be able to access each of them from time to time. However, your dominant chakra is where your dharmic life will find its maximum potential. That is the chakra in which your unique psychological and spiritual endowment can realize its fullest expression. It is where you actualize what you are meant to be.

Sadly, your dominant chakra may not be the one in which you live much of the time. Socialization and conditioning shape your persona and often influence which of the seven chakras becomes dominant in the first part of your life—before you develop karmic consciousness and recognize that your actions circle you back into maya time and again, rather than advancing you toward wellness. Parents and society can mold you to live your first life out of an auxiliary chakra in order to meet the demands of adaptation.

The heart chakra governs compassion and caring attachment. Dependent people, for example, live primarily out of the ida nadi in the heart chakra. They typically have difficulty exerting personal power and authority, and project their authority and power drives onto a spouse or an employer. This creates a relationship problem with the carrier of the projection. In fact, the problem is not really between the dependent person and the projection carrier, but rather stems from the dependent person's unlived energy being projected onto the other party. The task is to become conscious of this tendency and reclaim the projected energy, living it out as fully and responsibly as possible.

The heart chakra may or may not be the dominant chakra of the dependant person. It may be the chakra most strongly developed by the outside forces that shaped his or her persona. In order to get into the central sushumna nadi of their dominant chakra, dependent people may have to make a detour through other, auxiliary chakras. This detour may involve withdrawing their projections, recognizing that they are permitting others to live that (projected) part of their potential for them. In this case, they have to discover how they surrender their power and voice to others, and then reclaim them by learning to speak their own truth and exercise power in their own right.

Symptoms of migraine headache and thyroid problems in women may be indicative of problems in the heart and head chakras. When a woman is stuck at the level of the heart chakra, the throat chakra compensates by asserting its presence in the form of thyroid problems; the head chakra of intelligence speaks via headaches. The therapeutic task for this woman is to honor the needs of the throat chakra by finding an assertive voice for her viewpoints and claiming the authority of her head chakra by developing and expressing her intellect. Often, a woman in this situation is able to do this only in the second half of life, after fulfilling her karmic and dharmic chores of rearing her family.

Heart problems in many professional women and men may indicate a blockage in the navel chakra of personal power—the fire of ambition may be excessive and the heart chakra may protest through cardiac symptoms and conditions. Professional men who are stranded in the navel chakra of power, control, and authority do not rise above it to the next level—the heart chakra of compassion and intimacy. For these men, healing involves honoring the heart chakra by getting in touch with their feelings of loving attachment, sometimes only after they have their first brush with death in a heart attack or another major medical problem that puts their striving and professional success in perspective. Many such men learn to value love feelings and relationships only after a medical catastrophe.

The developmental goal of Kundalini balancing is to make appropriate use of all six auxiliary chakras as needed to consolidate your dominant-chakra management. The auxiliary chakras then become consultants or advisors to your dominant chakra. However, if you ignore your auxiliary chakras, they become ferocious adversaries and create problems in the form of projections or medical or psychiatric conditions, or as complications piggy-backing on pre-existing illnesses.

Root Chakra—Survival and Security

The first, or root, chakra is situated in the perineum between the anus and the genitals. The ruler of the first chakra is Ganesha, the elephant-headed god, lord of all beginnings and remover of obstacles.

Developing trust and an internal sense of emotional and material security are the tasks and goals of the first chakra. When you have succeeded at these fundamental tasks, you act in harmony with the natural rhythms of your body and psyche, neither wasting energy nor polluting sensory awareness with overindulgence. You act wisely and with moderation, and are able to explore body and mind as vehicles of liberation from maya and its allure.

Each of the seven chakras involves three dimensions to which you must attend. First, you must acknowledge the archetype that presides over the chakra and heed the developmental mandate of the archetype. In the root chakra, the archetype of the Great Mother beckons you to struggle with the opposing tensions of abandonment/engulfment and establish a sense of basic trust in others, the world, and yourself. Absence of this trust is apparent in all forms

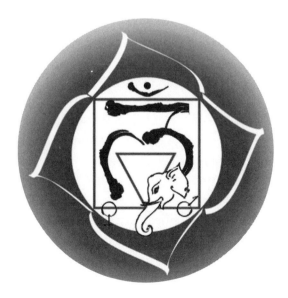

of schizophrenia, avoidant personality syndromes, and depression. Trust is dependent, not on sating your appetites or in exuberant demonstrations of love, but on the quality of the maternal relationship. The social dimension of trust is a touchstone of religion, with its childlike surrender to the universe. In centered individuals, religion is the path to *Unus Mundus*, access to the wisdom of the universe, and a sense of your place in the bigger picture.

You must also adjust any imbalance in the nadis. A preponderance of either masculine or feminine energy leads to imbalanced relationships. You must align with the central channel to integrate your masculine and feminine energies. If you are stuck in the feminine channel in the first chakra, you behave as the victim in a relationship; if you are stuck in the masculine channel, you behave as the aggressor. In such an imbalanced relationship, the goal of the two partners is to establish basic trust in each other, so that a dynamic of self-mothering and self-care can be established.

Finally, you must acknowledge any medical or psychiatric symptoms and trace them to the imbalance in the root chakra. Lower gastrointestinal problems are often symbolic of disturbances in the root chakra and must be attended to by developing trust and self-mothering. This moves the dynamic from the reptilian nervous system that is generating these symptoms, through limbic decoding of the Mother archetype issues in childhood, to a neocortical choice of more adequate self-mothering.

Eileen is a surgeon with severe chronic colitis that requires aggressive medical treatment, including long-term steroid use that caused complications of weight fluctuations, mood swings, and susceptibility to infection. Analytic treatment uncovered a cold, distant, emotionally unavailable mother who never acknowledged Eileen's considerable personal and professional success. By becoming a workaholic and constantly seeking love and affirmation from patients, peers, and family, Eileen acted as the Great Mother to all while failing to care for herself. This imbalance had to be corrected in therapy before healing could begin.

Pelvic Chakra—Generativity

The second chakra is called the *svadhisthna*—the "dwelling place of the self." It is located in the area of the hypogastrum and bladder, above the genitals. Its totem animal is the crocodile, which represents the serpentine, sensuous nature of people dominated by this chakra.

You must acknowledge the archetype of the Great Father as the gatekeeper at this synapse. The developmental task of the second chakra is generativity—both creative and procreative—and imbalance here can result in stagnation. While the attitude of the first chakra is single-minded and linear, fantasy and multiplicity enter the picture with the second chakra. Generativity implies gestating, nurturing your inner potential, and eventually giving birth to what has been developing inside you. In this sense, generativity is the capacity to parent yourself and your offspring using innate potential, talents, and skills. Here, the opposing tendencies of paternal control versus shame and doubt must be integrated in a balanced sense of autonomy through good self-parenting. This can begin with a teenager's wish to stand on his or her own two feet and

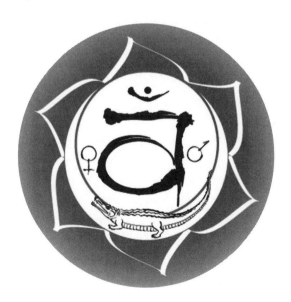

gradually make personal choices. By contrast, those in doubt or shame may attempt minute control of their environment or selves in an effort that can lead to obsessive neurosis.

Shame fosters a defense of invisibility for fear of being seen and ridiculed. Doubt is the brother of shame. Shame emanates from feeling exposed; doubt has to do with consciousness of having a front and a back that is vulnerable to attack, which can foster paranoia. In society, the second-chakra dynamic is apparent in the Apollonian quest for justice and order.

In this chakra, you must balance the modes of the masculine Exploiter and the feminine Martyr. Many people dealing with second-chakra problems are preoccupied with self-creation rather than with true relationships. They tend to recruit other people as sexual partners who function as vehicles for propagating themselves. Their relationships are frequently unsatisfying, shallow, or exploitative, and often end in tumultuous break-ups.

People stuck in either the second chakra's cool ida channel or the hot pingala channel identify the conscious part of their psyches as the Exploiter (pingala) or the Martyr (ida) archetypes. Identification with either role results in projecting the complementary role onto another person in their lives. Those in the Martyr role feel helpless vis-à-vis the Exploiter, while those in the Exploiter role feel contempt for the exploited (but they also feel unconscious guilt). When martyr and exploiter take back their projections, they can realign the imbalance, moving their energy into the central channel (sushumna nadi). Then they can become authentically generative in their endeavors, whether at work, in relationships, or at play. In other words, they experience themselves as parents to their inner potential and are compassionate but firm.

For people caught in the Martyr/Exploiter mode in the second chakra to attain pleasure, they must return to the first chakra and work on their unresolved survival issues. This may involve grounding themselves in basic life skills, establishing trust in place of exploitation as a mode of relating, and ascending to the third chakra of autonomy and self-control. If they can grow in these ways, they gain access to the pursuit of pleasure in its various forms and begin to actualize themselves and play useful roles in their communities.

You must attend to the medical and psychiatric symptoms that may be trying to draw your attention to second-chakra imbalance— prostate problems in men, and endometriosis and genitourinary-tract problems in women. When you address these issues, your symptoms can be relieved.

Robert consulted me for his obsessive personality and depression that developed along with prostate cancer. His father was controlling and shaming and always put him down. The only way Robert could get his attention was by becoming the troublemaker, the black sheep in the family. However, behind a rebellious persona lay a self-doubting individual who had exploitative relationships with women as a way to boost his self-esteem. His therapy involved gradual reclamation of his authentic creativity and talent. As he moved from self-doubt and shame to self-assertion and autonomy, his business started to blossom. He started to re-parent his personal and professional life, and recommitted himself to his loving wife and his affiliation with his church.

Navel Chakra—Autonomy

The third chakra is called *manipura,* or "plenitude of jewels." Its location corresponds to the solar plexus, between the diaphragm and the navel. The totem animal of the third chakra is the ram, the steed of Agni, the fire god. The ram depicts the fiery, headstrong nature of the third-chakra person. Individuals dominated by the third chakra strive for personal power and recognition, sometimes at all costs. When experiencing shame, they work themselves into a rage and attempt to defend and protect their sense of self. Doubt and self-doubt are twin emotions. The psychological issues of the third chakra are autonomy versus shame and doubt, and control versus letting go.

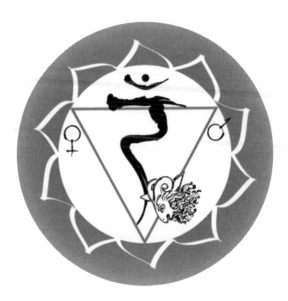

The first balancing act in the third chakra is to acknowledge the archetype of the Warrior or Hero. The Hero's journey of attack and conquest can be as simple as taking initiative in response to life's ordinary challenges and crises, as the child and adult aspects of your personality work through fear to grow together. The danger is that guilt can result from failing to meet goals, including the expectations of parents.

You must address the psychological drama of the navel chakra, which is focused on the dynamic of the Master (pingala nadi) and Slave (ida nadi) archetypes. Each of these roles is the shadow of the other; you can project them onto the important people in your life, creating difficulties with them. When caught in the dark side of the third chakra's maya, people feel a deep sense of shame in their role as Master or Slave. Once they become conscious of their projections, however, they have the possibility of taking them back. Integrating the projected characteristics into your personality balances the energy so that it flows in the sushumna, rather than in the pingala or the ida, nadi. You are then able to experience autonomy as well as connectedness when you enter into partnership with another person, rather than acting as that person's master or slave.

In the third chakra, the maya of controlling your work and relationships results in a Master/Slave karma. Since power excludes love, these relationships lack mutuality—you doubt the emotional availability of other people. Consequently, you often use shame or rage to control the people around you—whether employees, lovers, or children—if they do not comply with your wishes, which are often unstated or even unconscious.

People dominated by the third chakra must access the fourth-chakra energy of true mutuality, relationship, and intimacy with others so that they can use their fiery energy in a balanced and generative way to realize their selfhood and express their creative potential as individuals who contribute to the well-being of their families and their communities.

You must attend to the medical or psychiatric symptoms that are trying to draw your attention to the turbulence at this synapse. Patients with navel-chakra problems are often afflicted with stomach ulcers, colitis, or irritable bowel syndrome. These are signals from the reptilian nervous system of a limbic imbalance in the Warrior/Hero archetype. You must heal these problems neocortically by doing the inner and relationship work necessary to address the imbalance.

Roger is a well-established physician suffering symptoms of schizophrenia and depression. Gradually, he lost interest in his practice and eventually retired in his early fifties. Although he is a caring man, devoted to wife and family, Roger lived in his head and was unable to express his feelings. Before he fell prey to illness, he had been living out the Master dynamic of the third chakra. He was competent and intelligent, but ambitious and controlling, both in his profession and in his marriage, enslaving everyone by dazzling them with the fire of his authority and power. As he approached his fiftieth birthday, however, serious medical problems slowed his pace, and his devoted wife became depressed from carrying the feelings and emotions (heart chakra) for both of them. Roger was too intellectual to dabble in matters of the heart. The only way he could experience the fire of the third chakra was as intellectual excitement.

To heal, Roger had to re-establish his ability to feel by developing his heart chakra, enabling him to value his work emotionally. He was then able to reclaim the capacity to express feelings and have a consciously felt sense of devotion to his family.

To some extent, the depression component of his schizoaffective disorder put Roger in contact with a deep unconscious love (heart chakra) for his family that he had not been able to show previously. Gradually, Roger was able to claim his feelings and return to his primary third chakra so that he could meaningfully manage his available resources and remaining time in service to his selfhood and family.

Heart Chakra—Intimacy

The fourth chakra, called *anahata* or "unattackable," is located at the heart plexus behind the sternum. The heart chakra's totem animal is the deer or black antelope, both sensitive creatures full of inspiration.

The developmental task of the fourth chakra involves intimacy versus isolation. Just as the deer or antelope runs swiftly, often changing directions, the fourth-chakra person's emotions can fluctuate. Intimacy in the fourth chakra is based on feelings and the capacity to commit to affiliations and relationships while making the necessary sacrifices. The maya aspect of the fourth chakra is overdependence on relationships for self-esteem at the cost of autonomy and voicing your needs, values, and beliefs. The karma of the fourth chakra is either fear of isolation and abandonment, or codependency. To counter the fear of being abandoned, fourth-chakra people often preemptively withdraw from relationships. But when well managed, this chakra leads to positive relationships and provides the driving force to fulfill your responsibility to family and community.

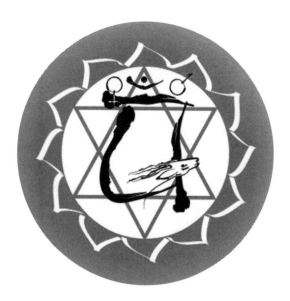

The first task in the fourth chakra is to pay respect to the Lover archetype that guides your relationships. You must reconcile the opposing tendencies of intimacy and isolation and establish the middle way of mutuality, which calls for compromise and sacrifice. Through this process, the self-involved sexuality of the second chakra evolves into the mutuality of the fourth.

Here, you address any relationship imbalance stemming from a lopsided identification with the masculine role of Caretaker or the feminine role of Dependent, and align your relationship with the central channel. When your fourth chakra is functioning optimally, you can both give and receive emotionally, and experience loving attachment, mutuality, and intimacy. In this chakra, predominance of either the pingala or the ida nadi leads to the Caretaker/Dependent dynamic and fears of emotional isolation or engulfment. Those dominated by the ida nadi often experience helpless dependency; those dominated by the pingala nadi are forced into the role of all-powerful caretaker. Each projects the other, unlived half of the Caretaker/Dependent split, which in turn creates relationship problems. If you are not careful, the need for intimacy and fear of isolation can lead to dependency and codependency.

When people integrate the projected missing half of the Caretaker/Dependent dynamic into their consciousness, they move into the central channel, the sushumna. This shifts their relationships out of the Caretaker/Dependent pattern, helping them feel like lovers rather than dependent parasites or overburdened caretakers. This leads to true intimacy rather than the emotional isolation of either the caretaker or the dependent. Buoyed by the gentle currents of intimacy, people feel they can truly love themselves as well as others. Problems result when you do not balance this dynamic. People dominated by the ida nadi manifestation of the fourth chakra can be trapped in codependency, while those stuck in the pingala nadi manifestation begin to deny all feelings and relational needs.

In this chakra, you must attend to the medical or psychiatric symptoms that are trying to draw attention to heart-chakra problems so that illness is not the primary channel of communication between your ego and your soul.

Mary has been married for many years to a man who does not communicate. Marty, her husband, was unable to express any feelings, and was stuck in a third-chakra power-and-control mode. Mary was an emotional person locked in a dependent relationship with her controlling husband. Mary and Marty shared a fourth-chakra problem.

Mary's natural primary chakra was the fourth. Since she was forced to do all the emotional caretaking in her marriage, however, her fourth-chakra pingala nadi worked overtime while Marty focused his energy on being a hero in his profession (pingala nadi dominating his third chakra). This relegated Mary to the third-chakra ida nadi, causing her to project her need for autonomy onto her professionally successful, but emotionally controlling, husband. In mid-life, Mary completed graduate school, but was unable to get much support from Marty to launch her long-cherished dream of a career. Consequently, she became clinically depressed and needed psychiatric intervention.

For his part, Marty projected his unlived dependency needs and unexpressed feelings onto his wife. Mary got caught in the Slave role of Marty's Master/Slave split and suffered the corresponding karma of isolation and depression. Marty, on the other hand, was trapped in the dependent side of the (fourth-chakra) Caretaker/Dependent dynamic, and finally suffered cardiac problems.

In the unconscious arrangement between Mary and Marty, Mary had always carried Marty's sad and dark feelings. The burden grew heavier as he faced professional reverses. He was no longer able to live out of his third chakra of autonomy and control as he lost his grip on his corporate milieu, nor was he able to depend unconsciously on Mary for emotional support. Thus, he became more and more disgruntled (and unconsciously depressed). Mary carried the depression for both of them in her fourth chakra of feelings.

This precarious balancing act finally broke down when Marty's mother died. He was unable to grieve and expressed no emotions. Feeling the grief for both of them, Mary got more depressed and even suicidal. The vicious cycle broke when Marty had a massive heart attack that forced him to let go of the illusion that he could control all professional and personal events in his life. Finally, forced to attend to his fourth (heart) chakra, Marty began to experience his emotions, and started to verbalize his grief over his mother's death and his hurt about professional reverses. He permitted himself to depend on Mary for love, nurturance, and emotional support, withdrawing some of the energy from his third-chakra pingala nadi and strengthening the ida nadi of his fourth chakra. He became open with Mary about his needs and their Master/Slave karma was retired. At long last, Mary and Marty became true partners and lovers.

For her part, Mary was able to move out of her third-chakra ida nadi into her third-chakra sushumna nadi of mastery and appropriate control. She began to shape her destiny and assert autonomy with Marty and her professional ambitions. For his part, Marty permitted himself the luxury of letting Mary take care of him in a new way as he expressed his fears and feelings about reverses and losses in his life. Gaining access to the feeling capacity of his fourth chakra, he recovered from his heart problems, mellowed in his aggressive pursuit of professional success, and became supportive of Mary's quest for autonomy. Mary has since found a good position in her chosen profession and is claiming her third chakra of autonomy and mastery in work and marriage.

Throat Chakra—Initiative

The fifth chakra—*vishudha,* or "purification" chakra—is situated in the throat at the pharyngeal plexus. With the fifth chakra, you move beyond physical reality into the realm of abstract ideas and the psyche. This is where you start to see events occurring, not only in their physical reality, but also on more subtle planes. The elephant is associated with the fifth chakra, a totem that stands for knowledge of nature and the environment, and that teaches patience, memory, and self-confidence.

A fifth-chakra person seeks only that knowledge that is timeless and true beyond the limitations of maya, culture, and conditioning. The main problem encountered in the fifth chakra is negative intellect, which occurs when individuals are cut off from the heart chakra and from the forehead chakra, which governs integrity and leadership.

In the fifth chakra, you must attend to the Trickster god, Hermes or Krishna. Developmentally, you must bridge the opposites of ego identity and ego confusion to achieve authentic self-expression— "finding your voice"—rather than merging your identity with that of your clan or nation, or some other group. People in whom the fifth chakra is optimally developed are intuitively perceptive, even clairvoyant, and able to communicate both verbally and non-verbally. They have found their own voices and can take the initiative

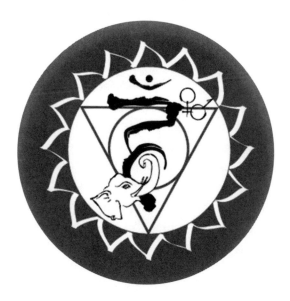

to express and live according to their own values, priorities, and beliefs. The voice of fifth-chakra people penetrates to the heart of the listener.

In the fifth chakra, you must attend to the relationship imbalance between the masculine Intimidator and the feminine Silent roles, centering these in your capacity to communicate with your own voice. The drama of the fifth chakra is between those who intimidate (dominated by the pingala nadi) and those who are intimidated and silent (dominated by the ida nadi). The drama plays out in a mutual unconscious projection in which each partner projects his or her opposite, unlived half onto the other. When the silent one and the intimidator take back their mutual projections, they (and their relationship) move to the central channel, where either person can take the initiative.

Medical and psychological problems of the fifth chakra manifest in the throat area, including thyroid problems. Men who over-advertise themselves develop narcissistic personality disorders; women may lose their authentic voice, expressing themselves only through their anxiety symptoms or fears of taking a personal or individual stand on issues.

In psychotherapy, Angie said: "I feel that my voice is not heard." The next week, she dreamed she was Ann Frank, writing in her dairy in a dark, desolate room. Angie feels alone and isolated—unheard by significant people in her life. The dream image accurately depicts her present life circumstances.

Angie is a successful professional in mid-life. Her grandparents immigrated to America prior to World War II. Many of her uncles and aunts perished in the concentration camps of Nazi Germany. Angie's childhood was turbulent, as her family struggled to integrate into American culture. Her father was overburdened at work and her mother was depressed and overwhelmed by the chores of parenting her family. Angie's parents grossly underplayed their rich ethnic roots to fit into what Angie calls the Gentile majority culture.

As the oldest child, the bulk of parenting responsibilities fell upon Angie. Although she had great potential to become a leader (her fifth chakra was the natural dominant), it was her maya to be stuck in the ida nadi of the fifth chakra as a silent caretaker. Consequently, she could not give voice to the emotions in her heart and exercise the initiative to pursue her own path.

Urged on by her chronic depressive symptoms and guided by her dreams, Angie gradually shifted energy to the sushumna nadi of her fifth chakra and became able to take initiative on her own behalf. This led to her being able to voice her values and priorities, to come out of hiding as a "closet Jew," and to claim her spiritual beliefs and worldview openly. By communicating her true values and beliefs, she became a source of inspiration for others, who find peace, calm, and understanding in her presence. Angie is no longer locked in the role of a voiceless caretaker of others.

Like Ann Frank, Angie is a courageous woman. No one listened to Ann Frank during her lifetime, yet her dairy became her voice and the immortal voice of oppressed people all over the planet. She became a living symbol for Angie, enabling her to reconnect with her spiritual roots and reclaim her rich heritage.

Eye Chakra—Integrity and Leadership

The sixth chakra—*ajna,* or "place of command"— is located between the eyebrows. Resembling the third eye or a winged seed, this chakra is the window to your inner vision. It allows you to see into your psyche, as well as into the transcendent world beyond the physical reality perceived by your two eyes. No animal form is associated with the sixth chakra, since its activity is perception of the non-material dimension of reality.

The psychological issues of the sixth chakra are ego integrity versus despair. You achieve ego integrity when you adapt to the trials, tribulations, and triumphs of your unique life journey and adequately fulfill this chakra's task, which is discovering where and how your particular existence meaningfully fulfills your relationship to your fellow human beings.

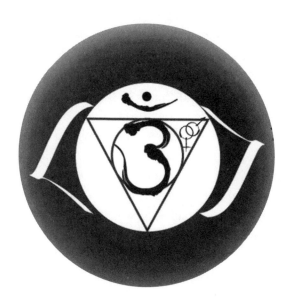

Psychologist Erik Erikson (Erikson, 1977) calls this stage of development "post-narcissistic self-love," the point at which you accept that your life journey has to be just the way it is in order to fulfill your svadharma. The labyrinthine, serpentine course of your individual life, with its trials and triumphs, then make sense and have meaning in the bigger picture of your community and times. Ego integrity leads to emotional and spiritual integration, permits meaningful and informed participation in your community, and enables you to assume leadership if called upon to do so.

The inner work of the sixth chakra begins with honoring the archetype of the Leader, who stands guard at this synapse. This archetype presents the opposing tendencies of generativity versus stagnation. Integrating these tendencies leads to leadership. With generativity, you can contribute to your family and community through productivity and creativity. You begin to see the world beyond the physical realm just as clearly as you perceive outer reality with your physical eyes. You recognize that individual existence is relative—part of a much larger mosaic of higher consciousness. Sixth-chakra people realize that they don't live life; rather, the larger design of nature lives them. They see their fragile, transient personal lives as precious pieces in the divine, cosmic rhythm of life. Sixth-chakra individuals are most readily able the ride the contours of destiny.

Integrity, one of the attributes of the sixth chakra, carries the connotations of conscience, incorruptibility, soundness, completeness, and honesty. The karmic task of people misusing the powers of the sixth chakra is to recognize their personal transience and insignificance. If they over-identify with the collective issues that live through them, they become inflated with narcissism. They resemble a bank teller who claims ownership of the sums of money passing through his hands rather seeing himself as the transient steward of this wealth. Their inability to maintain ego integrity while holding collective responsibility leads to despair, demoralization, and fragmentation of self—in a word, to existential depression, the despair and depletion resulting from not knowing your place or role on the stage of life and the world.

In the sixth chakra, you must balance the Leader/Follower split in your masculine/feminine modes of operating as it plays out in personal and community affairs. Here, the drama of Leader (in the hot pingala nadi) and Follower (in the cold ida nadi) manifests through mutual unconscious projections. Follower and leader both get caught in their respective mayas and project their tendencies onto each other. This sets up a society of few leaders and many followers; when leaders cannot deliver on their promises, these societies are plunged into despair.

Sooner or later, those who are locked compulsively in the leadership role fall from grace because they cannot fulfill all of their followers' expectations. This is inevitably the lot of false prophets and self-appointed gurus. Conversely, those who deny their potential for leadership, regardless of how limited it may be, set themselves up to resent the chosen or self-appointed leaders.

The karmic debt of followers who deny of their own leadership potential and of leaders who lack humility or are unwilling to surrender leadership when necessary creates imbalances within and between families, organizations, societies, and nations. When leaders and followers move into the sushumna nadi, they enter the realm of true participation in the affairs of the world, moving from the despair of fallen leaders and the resentment of followers to a state of empowerment that comes from informed, insightful participation. A sense of integrity develops. Now they are able to claim their rightful places in their communities and follow their own dharma.

In the sixth chakra, you must attend to the medical and psychiatric symptoms that call your attention to the eye chakra, especially migraines or other headaches.

Jody was in her fifties when she consulted me about her symptoms of depression, frequent headaches, and lack of intimacy with her husband, who had been inattentive for several years. Her emotionally distant father—a successful, hard-working businessman—had died the year before she started therapy, and Jody was still grieving his death. Consciously, Jody had seen her father as a man devoted to his family; unconsciously, however, she knew he had seldom been present for her and her siblings.

As I got to know Jody better, I saw that she tried to appear cheerful, accepting, and understanding of her situation. She worked hard at being a good mother and a good wife, but that actually meant that she did all the emotional work for everyone in her family. Underneath, I sensed a scared, dependent little girl who was afraid of men, as well as a powerful woman who could hold her own with anyone. Jody was carrying a lot of unlived life.

Jody's depression and headaches were related to two chakras. Like many women in American society, she had been groomed to do all the emotional work for the significant others in her life. This overworked her fourth (heart) chakra. When first meeting women like Jody, people often get the impression that their warmth, caring, and understanding are expressions of a dominant heart chakra. Sometimes this impression is correct; but often, their heart-chakra energy, while genuine, turns out to be a social adaptation—a fulfillment of society's expectations—and not the expression of their authentic dominant chakra.

For Jody, living from the heart chakra to the extent that she did had become a burden. She had had to carry, not only her own feelings, but also the unlived emotional life of her late father and emotionally unavailable husband. Her headaches were the protest of her sixth (head) chakra, telling her that she was not seeing the inner meaning of her overworked heart chakra and the depression it caused. Then, a series of seemingly chance events caught our attention.

Jody was very active in her suburban church. For some time, there had been talk of establishing a sister-church relationship with another congregation, but it had amounted to nothing more than well-intentioned talk. From time to time, Jody told me that her congregation's inaction frustrated her, but we did not pay much attention to the possible sister-church issue because it didn't seem to bear significantly on her depression, her headaches, or her suffering from her husband's emotional unavailability. Then in one session, Jody again mentioned the sister-church issue, and it occurred to me that perhaps there was more there than we had thought.

As I explored Jody's thoughts and feelings about a sister church in subsequent sessions, she brightened up. We were on to something. Jody realized that she really wanted her congregation to do something, not just talk about it. She offered to chair a committee to explore the needs of several inner-city churches and the possibilities for cooperation. As her committee got to work, Jody suffered from headaches less often. When she did experience a headache, we discovered that it started after she experienced frustration in her leadership role.

When Jody tapped her tremendous leadership qualities, her selfhood blossomed. As a leader in her church and community, her actions (karma) now serve the common good (varna dharma) rather than egotistical ends. She is realizing her dharmic potential.

Leaders who have navigated the path to the soul reach the realm of the sixth chakra of insight and leadership. When they are in the sushumna nadi of the sixth chakra, their leadership does not serve self-interest, but carries out God's work.

Crown Chakra—Spirituality and Moksha

The seventh chakra, the *sahasrara* chakra, is located above the crown of head. It is the place of Nirvana, where we are freed from all opposites—the realm where the individual soul and universal Spirit are one. In the realm of the seventh chakra, we are at one with nature, the collective psyche, and God, with no experience of the self as separate from God and nature. This is the reverse of the maya of the first chakra, where there is little awareness of nature as anything but an extension of ourselves.

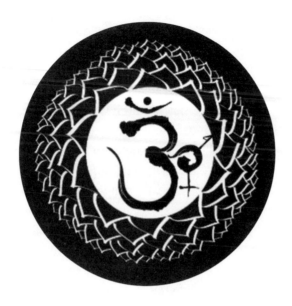

Some people in the seventh chakra are so lost in the collective psyche and the broader and deeper issues of life that they become divorced from outer reality. Trapped in the maya of the seventh chakra, they can fall prey to schizophrenia, and schizoid and schizotypal personality disorders. While they may have profound insight into the deepest questions and mysteries of human life, their insight is unusable for practical purposes and disconnects them from human encounters. The goal is to reconnect them with the outer realities of human life and the mundane issues of daily existence.

For this human contact, they have to consult and honor their first chakra (survival and security). When they balance the schizoid, autistic withdrawal of their seventh chakra with the karmic task of reconnecting with basic human concerns and relationships, they can fulfill their dharma and become authentic gurus, teachers, and mentors, guiding others on the path to higher consciousness. They can help the rest of us get a glimpse of the timeless mystery of our own existence in the greater plan of nature.

The guiding archetype of the seventh chakra is the Mentor, Guru, or Guide, which presents your consciousness with the opposites of ego integrity versus despair. The task for your consciousness is to bridge these with a spiritual attitude that grants you transcendent awareness of your place in the universe and enables you to guide others onto their path. Ego integrity is a stage in the ego's attainment of wisdom. It is post-narcissistic self-love—a sense of the self in service to Spirit, not the ego. It is awareness that the trials and triumphs of life have a pattern and meaning.

A common problem in the seventh chakra is an imbalance between the poles of narcissism and autism; when these are balanced, you gain the capacity to be a guide and a mentor, passing on the hard-earned wisdom of a lifetime. The drama of the seventh chakra plays out pathologically between two personality styles: the remote, withdrawn, seemingly other-worldly ascetic; and the narcissistic, self-aggrandizing, self-promoting person who claims to have a direct and exclusive connection to God. Locked in their respective mayic modes, withdrawn, emotionally inaccessible individuals are stuck in the cold ida nadi, while narcissists are locked in the hot pingala nadi. Each unconsciously projects the unlived half onto their opposites, who vicariously live it out for them. All too often, we see "spiritual leaders" and "gurus" fall from their pedestals as their clay feet crumble. These fallen idols have not been able to balance their energies in the pingala and sushumna nadis.

The crown chakra addresses the issues of reta dharma, the interface between the human and the divine. The dharma of individuals in the seventh chakra is to struggle with experiencing the meaning of human existence in the larger mystery of the cosmos. People with strong seventh chakras are attracted to metapsychological and theological pursuits.

When your seventh-chakra abode is informed and tempered by the first chakra (grounding in reality) and the sixth chakra (meaningful contact with community), you can live out its potential for spiritual pursuit grounded in reality and in service to community.

You can help humanity find itself and its place in the divine order of the cosmos. Gandhi, Christ, Buddha, and any priest or spiritual guide with integrity are all examples of this. They are old souls in their spiritual journeys who have the potential to achieve moksha—liberation from our human entanglement in maya and karma—and experience their oneness with the cosmos.

The final task in attaining balance in the crown chakra is to attend to medical and psychiatric symptoms that indicate turbulence at this synapse. Symptoms can include narcissism, autism, schizophrenia, headaches, and avoidant personality styles.

One of my patients, a priest with a deep sense of transcendence and of the mystery of life, could hardly function in the world. He is a good illustration of the dangers of getting lost in the seventh chakra.

When I first met Martin, I was awestruck. He seemed to dwell "on the mountaintop," with a deep sense of connection with God. But he was so disengaged from the outer world and from people that, despite his deep spiritual presence, he was unable to guide his flock. It was clear that he suffered from a kind of schizophrenia that isolated him from peers and parishioners alike. It was also apparent that Martin resided in the seventh chakra, where he experienced a deep sense of transcendence and the mystery of life. However, he was so preoccupied with these higher pursuits that he started to ignore the basic survival needs of his daily life. Deep in thought, he forgot to eat or leave his quarters for days.

Because he dwelled entirely in the ethereal realm of the seventh chakra, Martin's relationship to God became sterile. His experience of higher reality was not embodied in any tangible manner; his spiritual inflation cut him off from God's world. My psychotherapy with him focused on two major interventions. First, he had to get grounded in the first chakra of survival and reconnection with earth. With my guidance and prompting, Martin established a simple structure to deal with his daily survival needs. This included attention to meals, exercise, and contact with his mother and a friend.

For a while, Martin needed medications to ground him in his outer reality. As he integrated his first-chakra issues of survival with his sixth-chakra issues of community responsibility, he reclaimed his seat in the seventh chakra, tempered now and enriched by connection to his community of priests and parishioners and to his own human needs.

Balancing Your Kundalini

Use the following questions to gain insight into what you must do to achieve balance in your own chakras and in the flow of Kundalini through them:

- What are your dominant and auxiliary chakras?
- As you do your life-course chart of important events, illnesses, problems, relationships, goals, and pursuits to date, can you identify which chakras you have traveled through in your life? What did each of these chakra visits tell you about yourself?
- In which anatomical chakra location do you usually get medical or emotional symptoms? (For example, headaches for the seventh chakra, eye problems for the sixth chakra, throat problems in the fifth chakra, heart problems and depression for the fourth chakra, stomach problems for the third chakra, bladder and genital problems for the second chakra, and rectal, perineum, and emotional-security problems for the first chakra.)
- In your significant relationships, which chakra system is dominant? (For example, the Victim/Aggressor/Mother in the first chakra, the Martyr/Exploiter/Parent in second chakra, the Master/Slave/Partner in the third chakra, the Dependent/Caretaker/Lover in the fourth chakra, the Silent/Intimidator/Communicator

in the fifth chakra, the Leader/Follower/Participant in the sixth chakra, the Autistic/Narcissist/Guide in the seventh chakra.)

- What aspect of your life has activated your Kundalini experience? Is it your present life role, your medical or psychiatric illnesses, your life goals, your relationship problems, or some other aspect of your life experience?

- Based on your Kundalini understanding so far, what emotional and relational level have you achieved in each of the seven chakras?

- In balancing your root chakra, have you been able to heal the Aggressor/Victim relationship split into a self-caring paradigm? Have you been able to transcend abandonment/engulfment issues and establish a position of basic trust in yourself, others, and the world?

- In the second or pelvic chakra, have you been able to heal the Exploiter/Martyr relationship pattern into a self-parenting mode? Have you been able to transcend control, shame, and doubt and move into a sense of autonomy, generativity, and creativity?

- If you are a third-chakra person, have you recognized and healed your Master/Slave relationship pattern into a mode of partnership? Have you been able to transcend the dynamics of control and inferiority and establish a sense of initiative, enterprise, and mastery in life endeavors?

- If you are fourth-chakra dominant, have you recognized and integrated the Caretaker/Dependent relationship pattern and established a sense of mutuality in your relationships? Have you been able to transcend the tendency toward isolation and move toward a sense of intimacy and mutuality?

- If you are fifth-chakra dominant, have you recognized your Intimidator/Silent relationship pattern and established the mode of a communicator? Have you moved from a sense of confusion about your identity and found your own personal and professional identity and your authentic voice?

- If you are sixth-chakra dominant, have you identified your Leader/Follower relational patterns and established a participant mode of relationship? Have you moved from a sense of stagnation to leadership in your life?
- If you are seventh-chakra dominant, have you recognized your Narcissistic/Avoidant relational patterns and established a ground for mentoring others? Have you moved from a sense of despair about life and the future to a sense of your place in the bigger picture of your family, your community, and the world?

Chapter 5

Managing Your Personal Wellness Program

Once you have learned how to engage the Healing Zone and are familiar with some of the many methods for accessing it, the next stage is to create and manage your own personal wellness program. This is not meant to replace, but rather to supplement, any medical treatment you are currently receiving. Choose what feels right from the methods given above, then let your own intuition and feelings be your guide. If in doubt, consult your physician.

Setting Goals

The first step in establishing your own personal wellness program is to set goals. What do you hope to accomplish? Are you concerned about a specific medical or psychiatric problem? A relationship issue or a personality hang-up? The lack of joy or satisfaction in a certain area of your life? A desire for a higher level of vitality and engagement with life?

Personal Goals Questionnaire

Complete the questionnaire on the next page prior to starting your wellness program. Then revisit it weekly to track your progress.

Goals of Your Personal Wellness Program				
	No Problem	Mild	Moderate	Severe
Medical problem				
Psychiatric problem				
Addiction problem				
Relationship problem				
Personality hang-up				
Lack of feeling of well-being or satisfac-tion in life				
Other—List				

Emptying Your Cup

The next step is to empty your cup of illness and provoke behaviors that make room for wellness by recreating your consciousness with new images, energies, and potentials. While it may not be possible to empty your cup all at once or at the first attempt, you must be conscious of the importance of this task and proceed with baby steps—in small increments, one day at a time. You will gradually gain ground in your journey—a journey that calls for patience, perseverance, and persistence against the power of the dark side of your own nature. If you persist in this Hero's journey, the healing forces of the universe will step in to guide you on your path from illness to wellness.

Empty Cup Worksheet

Complete the following worksheet by checking off which of the behaviors or symptoms you need to target.

☐ Complexes, hang-ups

☐ Character defects—perfectionism, narcissism, histrionics, avoidance, self-defeating behavior, paranoia, withdrawal, intrusiveness, dependency

☐ Medical and psychiatric symptoms, obsessions, compulsions

☐ Addictive behaviors—alcohol, drugs, food, sexuality, gambling, the Internet, pornography

☐ Old grudges and resentments

☐ Grief over old losses

☐ Envy

☐ Dysfunctional attitudes and beliefs

☐ Dysfunctional attachments; enmeshed and dysfunctional relationships

☐ Codependency on another for self-esteem regulation

☐ Goals that have outlived their purpose in your life

The Circle of Life

The third step is to establish balance between love, work, play, and creativity in the circle of your life. People who are balanced in this way make us feel good and energized when we are in their presence. Imbalanced individuals drain our energy and vitality. Stick with the winners and aspire to be one.

There are many dimensions to this balance. You must balance experience with observation, introversion with extroversion, thinking with feeling, intuition with attention to detail, your tendency to take action with your capacity to reflect before you act. Your perception of apparent reality must be balanced by evaluating your thoughts and feelings before you act. Mundane concerns must be measured against reverence and respect for the sacred.

Life is not possible without balance; even your blood must be balanced within a very narrow range of pH (7.35–7.45). Anything above the range is alkalosis; anything below it is acidic. Without balance, you become stuck in the illness mode; with balance you can cross the Healing Zone into wellness. This may take time and require changes in your lifestyle. A spiritual attitude is the matrix of the Healing Zone.

Balancing Your Circle of Life

Complete the following circle as it represents your life sectors and compare it with the balanced circle of a winner. Monitor this on a weekly basis.

- First, divide this circle into four parts to represent the percentage of time you devote to love (relationships), work, play, and creativity.

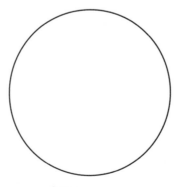

- Compare your circle with the ideal pattern shown here:

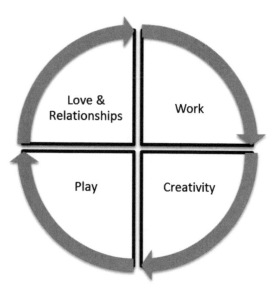

Finding Your Center

Now that you have listed your wellness goals and started to empty your cup of dysfunctional behaviors and attitudes, you must center yourself so that you can engage the Healing Zone. Your outer ego consciousness is a monkey mind that jumps from one branch to another, easily distracted by fleeting things. Centering is a personal spiritual practice to help yoke your ego consciousness to your deeper center—your soul.

Every religious and spiritual tradition has its own unique rituals to help seekers on a path to centering. As a therapist, my purpose is to help individuals evolve an individualized approach to engage their own centers amid the hustle and bustle of everyday life. The methods outlined in this book offer many other options to help you center yourself so you can safely navigate the Healing Zone and harvest its gifts.

For some, it may be easier to focus on pranayama or yoga; for others, meditation or music may act as a portal to wellness. Most find that daily journaling, dream recording, and mindfulness in attitude and practice are helpful. If you have access to guidance from a qualified practitioner, neurofeedback may be an excellent adjunct to your wellness program. Once you establish this program, stick with it for at least ten weeks and it will gradually become a part of your routine—like milk and honey.

Centering Questionnaire

Choose one or more of the following methods, and indicate the frequency with which you will pursue them.

Method	Daily	Three times a week	Weekly
Googling the unconscious			
Dream work			
Active imagina-tion			
Exploring fascinations and antipathies			
Recognizing complexes and hang-ups			
Resetting cog-nitive distor-tions			
Pranayama			
Yoga			
Meditation			
Mindfuness			
Music playlists			
Yantra drawing			

Method	Daily	Three times a week	Weekly
Kundalini balancing			
Journaling			
Centering prayer			

Engaging Your Triune Brain

While contemporary psychiatry and psychology have focused on the neocortical processes and Jungian psychology has made substantial strides in decoding the limbic archetypal strata of human consciousness, the ancients in India went deeper into the core autonomic reptilian strata of human consciousness and its essential role in healing illness and engaging our highest potential. The Indian healing traditions did not ignore the limbic and neocortical systems, but they proactively engaged the reptilian autonomic system. Western allopathic medicine has only recently begun to pay attention to these core strata of healing.

Throughout this book, we have discussed practical methods for engaging the wisdom of these three brains, with special emphasis on the autonomic nervous system. At a recent meeting of the American Psychiatric Association, I was heartened to see that mainstream American psychiatry is starting to pay attention to the role of autonomic instability in medical and psychiatric illness and treatment. At their annual meeting in San Francisco in 2009, Lawson Wulsin from the University of Cincinnati presented his research findings on autonomic imbalance and its role in depression and coronary artery disease (Wulsin, 2009).

Wulsin outlined several measures to monitor a person's autonomic health status, including measuring the resting heart rate, heart-rate variability, heart-rate recovery after exercise, and heart-rate turbulence (Srinivasan, 2006). Autonomic imbalances manifest in high sympathetic and low parasympathetic tones, leading to loss of the vagal inhibitory, or soothing, mechanism. A person who is out of balance is riding a runaway train. According to Wulsin (2009), autonomic imbalance may be a common pathway to illness and mortality. This certainly has been the view of ancient Indian healing practitioners.

The health of your limbic brain is manifest in your attention to the personal myth or archetype that guides your life journey. In the section on archetypes, I outlined some of the myths that guide us in the Healing Zone. Choose the myth best suited for your personal journey at the present time. For some, it may be necessary to honor the void of goddess Aditi; for others, it may be Bardo—the death of a certain dysfunctional aspect of their lives. Many find the guidance of Ganesha helpful in making auspicious new beginnings. Some may find the archetype of the transitional zone of the Lion Man helpful and use the practices that engage this zone—e.g., meditation. When caught in tight spots, at crossroads, or in the dilemmas of life, the guidance of the divine Trickster, Hermes, is invaluable.

The health of the neocortical brain is accessed by challenging your cognitive distortions, replacing them with rational thoughts, and invoking the ego functions of suppression, altruism, anticipation, sublimation, humor, reflective function, and a symbolic attitude.

Chapter 6

The Healing Zone—
Its Dark Side and Its Promise

There is no day without night. Light and shadow are two sides of the same coin. And the fourth level of consciousness also has its shadow side. Immersion in the energy flow of the universe in a systematic and respectful way, with reverence and skill, brings you handsome dividends of healing. However, there are those who force the hand of the universe by trying to make it give answers without adequate preparation, reverence, or follow-through on the guidance they receive. This arrogant and irresponsible attitude toward the universe and its consciousness can have disastrous consequences for these individuals and their families, and for society.

Gambling addicts are a common example of those who abuse the universe in this way. For the brief moment when the dice are rolling, they are connected to the flow of the universe. Tossing the dice brings an intense feeling that is ecstatic and freeing—a high that comes from connection with higher forces and the mystery of existence. This intensity of feeling becomes addictive, however; after a while, gamblers no longer play to win or lose, but rather to experience this reckless connection with this energy. They are caught in the flow and swept away into the dark abyss of the psyche.

If you roll the dice to get a response to a serious question that your outer consciousness is unable to resolve, however, the universe will guide you—if you know how to interpret the response. Through dice, the universe speaks in a language of the unconscious that must be decoded using the symbolic systems of ancient traditions. The *I Ching* is one such method. By casting coins or using similar methods, you can ask the universe serious questions and it will give you detailed and helpful answers.

The Healing Zone holds three other perils as well. Some get too comfortable with the void; some compulsively try to avoid it in a compensatory manner; others are seduced by the energy of the new creation and emerging consciousness, and become addicted to that sensation.

For those who become too comfortable with the void, there is a danger of falling into a depressed, dysthymic mode of adaptation. Clinically, these individuals suffer from chronic low-level depression, low energy, social withdrawal, lack of initiative, lack of drive, and an overly reflective attitude that becomes a defense against engagement with life. Others present avoidant personality traits, defined by the American Psychiatric Association in its diagnostic manual as a "pervasive pattern of social inhibition, feelings of inadequacy, and hypersensitivity to negative evaluation."

On the other hand, there are people who are so fearful of experiencing the void that they compensate for it by compulsive avoidance behaviors, including addiction to alcohol and other drugs, food, sex, gambling, and pornography. Even more serious are codependent relationships in which individuals avoid the dark experience of the void by living their lives vicariously through another individual—a spouse, children, or a lover. One benign-looking, but potentially malignant, addiction is a compulsive preoccupation with the Internet. I have met patients whose mindless online grazing is a time-consuming addiction harmful to their personal and professional lives.

For others addicted to the creation of a new consciousness in the Healing Zone, problems may involve hypomanic states and attention-deficit and hyperactivity disorders. Hypomania is an elevated mood that manifests in symptoms like rapid speech, inflated self-esteem or grandiosity, decreased need for sleep, racing thoughts, easy distractibility and attention deficit, and involvement in pleasurable activities that may have a high potential for negative psychosocial or physical consequences—unrestrained buying sprees, reckless driving, sexual indiscretions, or foolish business investments (Gartner, 2005). Some people in this state may seem unusually cold, uncaring, or arrogant, showing little or no emotional responsiveness.

People in hypomanic episodes do not have delusions or hallucinations. They do not lose touch with reality, in the sense that they know who they are and what is real. What can be a problem, however, is that they tend to overestimate their capabilities and fail to see the obvious risks involved in their ventures. Another common danger is that individuals can get so seduced by experiencing the void that they become tourists on the journey rather than settling in and consolidating their new insights. They become seekers rather than doers.

Finally, others short-circuit the process of seeking and consolidating the Healing Zone through drugs or mind-altering substances. Although this may give them transient access to the Healing Zone, it is like giving a sharp knife to a child rather than a skilled surgeon. Usually, these novices harm their minds, bodies, relationships, and souls through the careless use of drugs.

While there are perils in the Healing Zone, however, it offers hope and promise for a new beginning in 21st-century mind/body medicine, since it is both informed by the past and ready for the future. The new psychology of the Healing Zone connects the past, present, and future of medicine and emerging healing paradigms into a quantum reality of fundamental transformation. Contemporary physicians, therapists, and healers must transcend the mind/body/soul/Spirit/nature split and think of individuals in their present state of health as the current readout of their program of existence. In other words, what we see today in any individual is merely the present page in the book of his or her life, not the whole book. When you become curious about the rest of your own book—your own life story—you can access the potential of deep healing and the purposeful alignment of the present page and chapter with the rest of the story.

The Healing Zone of consciousness involves an exploration

of the spiritual dimension of wellness. Your wellness comes from following your purpose in this lifetime. Your illnesses come from misalignment with your spiritual purpose. This book offers some emerging paradigms for the journey from illness to wellness, focusing on the healing states of consciousness that bridge the synapses of the mind, body, soul, and Spirit, using ancient archetypal guidance to help you treat your problems and fulfill your potential. The methods offered here have been tried out in the trenches treating depression, addiction, and other maladies of the mind, body, and soul over the last thirty-five years of my clinical practice. However, they are based on 5000 years of Eastern healing tradition and two million years of ancestral wisdom that is encoded in the limbic brain.

This vast source of guidance and wisdom is available for you to explore. It can guide you in crisis and trauma, initiations and transitions, development and change at every crossroad of your life. You only have to access it. You may ignore it at your own peril—or you can engage it to fulfill your destiny. The choice is yours.

Every great tradition on our small and fragile planet offers us a path to this source. When you engage your own tradition—whether Hinduism, Islam, Judaism, Christianity, Buddhism, animism, or personal spirituality—you can exponentially deepen the healing impact of your efforts. Sadly, we often spend time negating the traditions of others rather than developing the potential for collaboration. There is enough human suffering already, and no one tradition has all the answers. We need each other to attend to human suffering and the human condition.

Emerging science—including quantum physics, genomic mapping, triune-brain research, archetypal understanding, neuroimaging, scientific study of meditative and mindfulness states, and exploration of the neuroplastic impact of psychotherapy—throws new light on the spiritual traditions of different cultures. If we can suspend our biases and prejudices, there is much we can learn from each other for the collective good.

Science points the way to hope and Spirit. Whenever we explore the spiritual, it leads to scientific insights. However, when we go to the core of science, it merges into spiritual wisdom, creating a transcendent zone of human consciousness and universal wisdom. While we should establish partnership between the two, we must acknowledge that, in the end, all science will fade into the mist of Spirit. It is the mystery of Spirit that creates the illusion of life and death, health and illness, grief and bliss. These are fleeting states. It is Spirit that endures. When we accept this with humility, we tune in to the healing wisdom of the universe and emerge from illness into wellness.

Appendix:

Physics and the Psyche

By Dr. Alkesh Punjabi–Director,
Center for Nuclear Fusion Research,
Hampton University

The field of quantum physics has illuminated the field of depth psychology in unexpected and fascinating ways. In fact, the ultra-quantitative discipline of physics has given us some illuminating insights into the workings and potential of the human psyche. Without getting lost in the daunting complexities of quantum theory, here are some of the things we have learned from it.

Oscillations are characterized by their frequency and wavelength—the higher the frequency, the higher the energy of oscillatory motion. Light is an electromagnetic oscillation. Different frequencies of electromagnetic oscillation appear to human eyes as different colors. In quantum mechanics, an object (like an electron or photon) manifests itself either as a wave or as a particle, depending on how an observer interacts with that object. The particle and wave manifestations of an object are mutually exclusive. But photon and electromagnetic oscillations are particle and wave manifestations of the same transcendent physical reality.

Gamma rays are electromagnetic oscillations of very high frequency. The energy of electromagnetic oscillations is given by the relation $E=h\upsilon$. E is energy; h is the constant of proportionality (called the Planck constant); υ is the frequency. A gamma ray's photon can spontaneously metamorphose into a pair—an electron and a positron—in a process called pair production. Electrons and positrons are anti-particles of each other. Sometimes an electron and a positron can annihilate each other and produce a gamma ray in a process called annihilation. For pair production to occur, however, it is necessary for the gamma rays to possess the minimum threshold energy, or the minimum frequency. So we can say that, when the frequency of electromagnetic oscillations (gamma rays) is above the threshold frequency, it can metamorphose and create a pair—a particle and its anti-particle.

Given sufficiently high frequency, gamma rays can thus transcend to a new state of being. By extension, when human brain-wave frequency crosses a certain threshold, the psyche can create a new state of being for itself. The physical and psychological situations are mathematically equivalent. Once a critical frequency is achieved, the system can spontaneously transform and transcend its state of being, and exist in a new state completely distinct from its old state.

When a large number of atoms or molecules in a region of space emit electromagnetic waves in lock step with exactly the same frequency, they create a laser beam (Light Amplification by the Stimulated Emission of Radiation). Lasers are coherent electromagnetic oscillations. They are very powerful and can focus extremely well. By extension, when a large number of neurons in the confines of a region of space called the brain collectively generate high-frequency waves with almost exactly the same frequency, the brain can transcend itself and, in that transcendental psychological space, focus on and illuminate an object in that space extremely well. When experienced meditators achieve a gamma frequency on their EEGs, they may be creating a new state of consciousness—a laser-sharp state of mindfulness.

It is well-known in physics that, if we cool a metal like copper close to absolute zero, we can make a superconductor. When a system is cooled, the random jiggling of its constituent molecules slows down, and the friction caused by the random jiggling of molecules in the free flow of electrons is diminished. At absolute zero, the random (undirected) motion of molecules completely stops, and electrons can flow without any resistance whatsoever. The flow of electrons is what causes electrical current in metals, and the unimpeded, free flow of electrons at absolute zero temperature creates a superconductor. Again by extension in psychological space, when the random wanderings of the human psyche are eliminated in the blissful state of meditation, the free unimpeded flow of psychological energy can constitute a "superconducting" of consciousness, allowing the Healing Zone to quell the turbulence in mind, body, and soul and restore a state of health, bliss, and wholeness.

Glossary

Active imagination. A technique developed by C. G. Jung in which you choose an image or a figure from a dream (for example), and engage it in a dialogue, just as you might a flesh-and-blood person. A guide is valuable when doing active imagination to help you relate the vivid images to the realities of your current life meaningfully. It is easy to make too much or too little of a picture, and either extreme overshoots the mark, causing you to lose the message in the exaggeration.

Ahimsa (*a* = lack of; *himsa* = violence). The principle of nonviolence as practiced by Gandhi, who prohibited physical, emotional, or spiritual violence against ourselves or our adversaries. You may confront the dark side of yourself or another, but only with love and an awareness of their humanity and underlying goodness.

Archetypes. Roles and patterns that are, so to speak, the natural laws or "dynamic skeletons" that structure our expectations and experiences. Archetypal patterns are subsets of the four aspects of dharma as well as of adharma, the shadow aspect of dharma. To put it another way, dharma and adharma actualize in typical ways that we can observe in life, literature, mythology, history, or any human activity. You can also think of archetypes as high-level sets of instructions. When an archetype is activated, the instructions in it organize what you see, how you feel, the way you depict it, and what you do. This process creates a perceptual/emotional/representational/behavioral mini-program that can operate in your psyche pretty much independently of your conscious choice and, if you are unaware of it operating in the background, assimilate ever more material to itself.

Ashrama dharma. The necessary developmental tasks of each of life's several stages—the calling to fulfill the responsibilities with which life presents us as we mature. Adolescence transforms the child; marriage and family transform the single young adult into parent and householder. When your children leave home and the nest is empty, you enter another developmental stage that calls you again to change and transform from parenting children to mentoring younger adults—often other people's children, or younger colleagues and co-workers. And as you look forward to your later decades, you become more concerned with the meaning of life and spiritual issues than with the day-to-day affairs of the world.

Atman. The individual soul; in Hindu terminology, a fractal of the Primal Soul, the *Brahman*. The individual soul is capable of spiritual and physical experience. It is both your window to the Primal Soul and the "organ" that registers the quality of your life. When your individual soul is afflicted, you suffer in various ways. Moreover, your connection to the Primal Soul is obscured, sometimes to the point that you need to be reminded vividly that there is any such thing as a soul connection.

Bardo. The Buddhist concept of "intermediate state," also translated as "transitional state," "in-between state," or "liminal state." Tibetan Buddhism postulates six Bardo states: the Bardo of this life, the Bardo of meditation, the Bardo of dreams, Chikka Bardo at the moment of death, Chonyid Bardo between death and rebirth, and Sidpa Bardo at the moment of rebirth. The term is often mentioned in the West in the context of Bardo Thodol. *Thodol* means "liberation," especially through hearing the funerary text of Tibetan Buddhism known as the *Tibetan Book of the Dead*.

Brahma. See Trimurti.

Chakras. In Hindu philosophy, the seven force centers located at particular points along the human body. Chakras are focal points for the reception and transmission of energy and can be accessed through the practice of Kundalini yoga. They are the synapses where the body, mind, soul, and Spirit manifest in interchangeable form.

Circumambulation. Literal or figurative circular motions that express the impulse or intention to define, relate to, approach, or protect the center and what is enclosed in the circle. This practice of encircling is an archetypal idea—that is, an idea that is ancient, that occurs in many cultures and times, and that has a powerful emotional effect on people. Circumambulation defines the boundaries of a sacred space by relating to a center of value, whether by meditating, by performing a sacred ritual, or by following the meander of your life. In the course of life, you gradually recognize that you have "circled around," thereby identifying and protecting certain central values many times.

Chaturvarga. The "four-fold good." Hindu ethics recognizes four pursuits that embrace everything a person can desire: pleasure (*kama*), wealth (*artha*), freedom (*moksha*), and a life in harmony with your inherent nature, your developmental stage, and your station in life, as well as with the Higher Power and the order of the universe (the four aspects of dharma, which is the sure guide for the other three).

Complex. Typical and normal features of the psyche that operate in the same way that the mind cross-references experiences in memory. Complexes are not fundamentally bad, but are rather emotional hot spots or hang-ups. When you have a complex—or a complex has you—your normal personality is taken over. Typically, you attempt to disown what just came through you—"I wasn't myself"; "I don't know what got into me." These hang-ups—technically known as "feeling-toned complexes"—get you into difficulties in your relation-ships and compromise your inner and outer adaptation.

Depression. One of the most frequent and painful psychiatric disor-ders. It can be treated aggressively by both medication and psycho-therapy. However, therapists and patients alike consistently bypass the soul-healing aspects of depression. Depression is often a messenger of the soul that arrives with the script for re-establishing balance and wholeness in life. Medical and psychiatric conditions are Janus-faced; they look both to the past and to the future.

Dharma. The "timeless order of nature," the archetypal patterns and natural laws. Dharma has four principal aspects, or archetypal dimen-sions, ranging from the individual to the cosmic. These are *svadharma* (the law of your own being, the individual uniqueness that strives for actualization within the context of your family and society, and your place and time in history); *ashrama dharma* (the stages of life with their various culturally shaped archetypal patterns to fulfill and their attendant responsibilities); *varna dharma* (the typical patterns of behavior, attitude, and emotion of your species); and *reta dharma* (universal spiritual and physical laws). These aspects represent the four spiritual purposes in your life: realizing your self-potential (*svadharma*), attending to your family (*ashrama dharma*), altruistic participation in community affairs (*varana dharma*), and pondering your connection with the divine intention (*reta dharma*). Your life can be out of dharmic balance—an excess here, a deficit there. When this is the case, the principle governing your adaptation to outer circumstances and the inner necessities of dynamic homeostasis and self-actualization attempt to restore equilibrium.

Individuation. Coming into selfhood or self-realization. This is the powerful force in each of us that propels us to actualize our unique psychological reality consciously—including our strengths and our weaknesses. Ultimately, individuation leads to the experience of a transpersonal regulating authority as the center of your individual psyche. It gives you a sense of being part of the whole—a fractal of the bigger picture of the collective purpose of this world.

Kama. A Hindu concept that addresses the experiential dimension of life: pleasure, love, and enjoyment. The pleasure that encourages relationships, fosters procreation and new life, forges attachments, and ensures the continuation of the species. Earthly love, sexual love, the pleasures of the world, aesthetic and cultural fulfillment, the joys of family and friends, and intellectual satisfaction all find their place in kama—a concept that is foreign to much of the Christian tradition. Hinduism does not make pleasure the highest good, but acknowledges that there is nothing wrong with pleasure and seeking it, as long as you obey the basic rules of morality—don't cheat; don't steal; don't lie; don't succumb to addictions. Kama also embraces the satisfactions and enjoyment of happiness, security, creativity, usefulness, and inspiration.

Karma. Sanskrit word meaning "action." The law of karma implies that the universe is an eternal moral order. Behind the apparently blind mechanical forces governing the cosmos, there exists a cosmic intelligence, a power that controls the operations of nature and guides the destiny of humankind. Karma emphasizes the freedom of human choice. By the choices you make today, you retire the consequences of past actions and lay the foundation for the future.

Karmic complexes. The psychic/somatic units into which your emotional experience is organized. These are the functional units localized in the chakras that have arisen through the interplay of maya, karma, and dharma. The core around which a karmic complex takes shape is a typical human situation—an inherent, archetypal pattern ready to organize your perceptions, your emotions, your imagery, and your behavior in a typically human way. Karmic complexes are archetypes in their structured, incarnated form. The archetypal patterns informing them organize behavior, perception, representation, and emotion. These four dimensions are interrelated. Your karmic complexes can either lead you into more karmic entanglements or serve as stepping-stones toward dharma. It's up to you which path you tread.

Kosha. Sanskrit word for "sheath." In Indian healing systems, the term refers to each of the five coverings of the Atman, or soul, which represent a holistic system encompassing the nature of being human. These include the physical or gross body, the breath or energy body, the emotional body, the intellectual body, and the bliss body. The Atman is considered the causal body, while the bliss, intellectual, emotional, and breath bodies constitute the subtle body. The physical body is the gross body.

Laxmi. See Trimurti.

Mandala. A sacred symbol consisting of archetypal forms enclosed in a circle. In Hinduism and Buddhism, mandalas are often used as a focus for meditation. Jung considered them as symbols of the self and the soul. What you depict in the mandalas you draw, he claimed, is an X-ray of your soul at that point in time.

Maya. A word often translated as "illusion." This is misleading, however. Of the several meanings embraced by the term, perhaps the fundamental sense is the cosmic creative force that generates concrete worlds, as well as the captivating nature of what is created, which binds souls.

Moksha. Liberation in the form of caring detachment. All individuals have the potential to achieve liberation from the misery of the human condition and the repetitive cycles of maya and karma. Moksha comes through the fulfillment of artha and kama (*chaturvarga*) under the guidance of dharma. In other words, when you have lived life to the full, and have actualized your innate potentials, your desire for artha and kama (wealth and pleasure in their various forms) no longer drives you. You are no longer attached to worldly joys or sorrows. This does not mean, however, that you have become indifferent. Moksha is detachment from the outcome, *not* from engagement in the enterprise, since to fulfill life, you must live it as duty to Spirit and to God, however you may conceive that higher power.

Nadis. The three channels through which subtle energy moves through the chakras. Two of the nadis (pingala and ida) correspond to the sympathetic and the parasympathetic nervous systems. Kundalini flowing primarily in one or the other of these nadis results in an energy imbalance that correlates to Type-A and Type-B personalities. The desirable condition is for neither to dominate, but rather for the energy to flow naturally and in a balanced way in the third nadi, the central channel called the sushumna nadi.

Neurofeedback (EEG feedback). A technique enabling you to alter your brain waves. It uses electroencephalographic (EEG) recordings of the brain waves to reset your brain-wave patterns to a more optimal frequency. It is used for many conditions and disabilities in which the brain is not working as well as it might. Neurofeedback helps control mood disorders like anxiety and depression, and can treat problems with the central nervous system like conduct disorder, temper tantrums, specific learning disabilities or ADHD, sleep disorders, epilepsy, and cognitive dysfunction resulting from head trauma, stroke, or aging. It is also used for patients undergoing cancer treatment to reduce stress, pain, and nausea, and to enhance immunity.

Persona. A term Jung uses to designate all the skills that constitute your function of adaptation to the outer world—your "outer" face. Your persona usually differs to a greater or lesser extent from your real individuality and authentic self, especially in the first life when maya dominates your consciousness. As you develop the persona you have chosen (or that has been chosen for you by your social environment), you neglect substantial aspects of your possibilities, thereby creating your "shadow."

Projection. An activated complex that overlays a present situation. Projection differs from blaming. When you blame, you do so intentionally. By contrast, you do not deliberately project. Projections happen when someone or some situation resembles another person or experience around which a karmic complex has formed, and you do not recognize the difference between what you are seeing now and what you saw and experienced in the past.

Reta dharma. The calling of the divine principle and law underlying all things. At the level of the human individual, reta dharma is the archetypal drive to relate to a higher power. You can think of reta dharma as honoring the transpersonal powers that move in you by giving appropriate expression to those powers. We each do this in our own unique way, in accord with our own svadharma, and in the context of our ashrama dharma and our varna dharma. In other words, spirituality and caring for the soul are part and parcel of being human.

Sarasvati. See Trimurti.

Satyagraha (*satya* = truth; *agraha* = insistence). The principal of the pursuit of and insistence on truth at any cost. Eventually, this became the cornerstone of contemporary Indian philosophy as *Satya Mave Jayate* (Hail the truth).

Shadow. In the broadest sense, all of your unlived life—both "good" and "bad." Your shadow includes all the relatively inferior parts of your personality, which are often transparent to those who know you well, though you may not be aware of them consciously or may wish not to be so. The shadow is a real live force in the psyche with, so to speak, a mind of its own. Sometimes, your shadow can take over and live through you. When that happens, you typically say: "I wasn't myself," or "I don't know what got into me." Remember, however, that your shadow also holds much unlived life—perhaps even your greatest gifts—which, for one reason or another, you have not cultivated.

Shiva. See Trimurti.

Shakti. See Trimurti.

Shiva/Shakti. Spiritual force that presides over the creation of a spiritual attitude that can lead to a new order—a new/renewed life after the destruction of the old. The mystery of Shiva/Shakti is that destruction *always* holds the potential and promise to renew life and remove the obstacles that keep you from actualizing your spiritual potential. You can, for example, view the painful consequences of your choices as Shiva/Shakti trampling you underfoot. You can learn to see other people who confront you and force you to look at yourself and your actions as Shiva/Shakti's agents. Or you may have a dream that shows something being destroyed.

Symbol (symptom). The best possible expression for something otherwise unknown to you. Something whose meaning or reference is fully known—like the red octagon bearing the word "Stop"—is not a symbol, but a sign. An image becomes a symbol for you only when you find it fascinating and meaningful, even though you are at a loss to say what the unexpressed meaning is. In this sense, a person to whom you have a powerful emotional response or reaction for which you cannot account may be a symbol. In other words, the carrier of your projection (of a part of yourself you don't recognize) is, for you, the best possible representation of that unknown aspect of yourself.

Synchronistic events. Coincidences that cannot be explained by causality; meaningful coincidences that we notice. The soul arranges synchronistic events to draw your attention to a constellation of energies, events, people, and circumstances in such a way that some aspect of your soul potential can be embodied in your life at that moment—a kind of "Heads up!" urging you to pay attention. These are mysterious and sacred moments when cosmic forces, your soul energy, and events and people in your outer life are in optimal alignment for some invisible aspect of your soul to become visible—if only you acknowledge them, attend to them, and act upon them in a conscious manner. Synchronistic events are evidence of a close connection between the two or more parties or things involved.

Svadharma. The calling to honor and actualize your individual uniqueness. The first lesson that maya and karma teach has to do with your innate, individual pattern, which finds expression in your particular physical, mental, and emotional nature. You can realize the other three dharmas only through being what you actually are. Hence svadharma is dharma individualized. Within the limits set and the challenges posed by your svadharma, you fulfill the other three dharmas.

Triune brain. A model of the evolution of the human brain proposed by American physician and neuroscientist Paul D. MacLean. The triune brain consists of the reptilian, the limbic, and the neocortical brains, which are viewed as structures sequentially added to the forebrain in the course of evolution. The reptilian brain is responsible for innate, stereotyped, species-typical behavioral patterns necessary for survival. The limbic system is responsible for enhanced emotion and motivation, as well as enhanced learning and memory. The neocortical brain is concerned primarily with what is happening in the external world. In humans, it is also responsible for language, planning, introspection, and self-awareness (consciousness).

Trimurti. The Hindu trinity composed of Brahma/Saraswati, Vishnu/Laxmi, and Shiva/Shakti. The function of Brahma/Saraswati, the universal force in its aspect as creator, is to bring multiplicity into being in place of the Primal Unity. Thus it is Brahma who creates maya, the limited or relative realities in which we actually live on earth. He does this in collaboration with his consort, Saraswati, the goddess of knowledge, arts, academic pursuits, and truth. Creative enterprise remains uninformed and ungrounded if Saraswati is not honored.

Turiya. In Hinduism, the experience of pure consciousness, rather than a state of consciousness. We live in three states of consciousness: waking, sleeping, and dreaming. Turiya is the fourth state of consciousness that bridges the other three, as well as the background underlying them. In Hinduism, it is also referred to as *chaturtha,* or the fourth state of consciousness.

Varna dharma. The "law of your kind" that calls you to fulfill your responsibilities to community. It defines your archetypal and socially determined interpersonal responsibilities within family, community, class, occupation, society, and nation.

Vishnu. See Trimurti.

Vishnu/Laxmi. The cohesive force that maintains the continuity of existence and the timeless order of nature that interconnects all that exists—thus called the "All Pervasive," "The Preserver." Laxmi is the patron goddess of wealth, prosperity, and peace, the prerequisites for maintaining the order of dharma in the world. Vishnu reincarnates in one of his several forms (avatars) to reestablish the timeless order whenever necessary. Vishnu/Laxmi can work through the sage and time-tested advice your friends may give you.

Yantra. Sanskrit for "instrument" or "machine." In the context of spirituality or meditation, a yantra is a symbol constructed from geometric forms used to balance the mind or focus on spiritual concepts. It uses the concepts of sacred geometry to engage the spiritual forces of the universe for health and healing. Your body is also a yantra with its own sacred geometry that engages the spiritual forces of the universe when you attend to it with wisdom, knowledge, guidance, and reverence.

The construction of different yantras activates corresponding archetypal energies to guide you onto the path to the soul.

Yoga. A term meaning to "yoke," to "join together." Kundalini yoga aims to integrate your individual consciousness with dharmic consciousness, your individual soul with the Great Soul. In yoga, as in all attempts to mature and grow emotionally and spiritually, you must cultivate moral preliminaries—non-injury (ahimsa), truthfulness, self-control, the discipline to scrutinize yourself, and the desire to reach your goal.

Bibliography

Alper, M. (2008). *The "God" Part of the Brain: A Scientific Interpretation of Human Spirituality and God*, Sourcebooks, Inc.

Antonova, I., E. R. Kandel, and R. D. Hawkins (2003). "Activity-dependent presynaptic facilitation and Hebbian LTP are both required and interact during classical conditioning in Aplysia," *Neuron*, January 9.

Avalon, Arthur (Sir John Woodruff) (1918). *Shakti and Shâkta, Essays and Addresses on the Shâkta Tantrashâstra*, Luzac & Co.

Baehr, E. et. al. (1999). "Clinical Use of an Alpha Asymmetry Neurofeedback Protocol in the treatment of Mood Disorders," in *Introduction to Quantitative EEG and Neurofeedback*, Academic Press.

Beck, Aaron T. 1980; 1979. *Cognitive Therapy of Depression*. Chichester: Wiley.

Bedi, Ashok (2000). *Path to the Soul*, Samuel Weiser Inc.

————— (2007). *Awaken the Slumbering Goddess: The Latent Code of the Hindu Goddess Archetypes*, Booksurge Publishers.

Bedi, Ashok and Boris Matthews (2003). *Retire Your Family Karma*, Nicholas-Hayes.

Benson, Herbert (1975). *The Relaxation Response*, William Morrow and Company, Inc.

Berk, T. S. (1989). "Neuroendocrine and stress hormone changes during mirthful laughter," *American Journal of Medical Science*, 298, 390–396.

Bruhn, S. W. (1998). *The Power of Clan: The Influence of Human Relationships on Heart Disease,* Transaction Publishers.

Burke, W. J. and F. A. Moreno (2006). "Suicidality and Treatment Resistant Depression: Results from a Twenty-Four-Month Trial of Vagus Nerve Stimulation," presented at the 156th American Psychiatric Association annual meeting, May 20–25, Toronto.

Cahn, B. Rael and John Polich (2006). "Meditation States and Traits: EEG, ERP, and Neuroimaging Studies," *Psychological Bulletin*, 132: 2.

Cannon, W. B. (1915). "Bodily Changes in Pain, Hunger, Fear and Rage: An Account of Recent Researches into the Function of Emotional Excitement," Appleton.

Chopra, Deepak (1990). *Quantum Healing—Exploring the Frontiers of Mind/Body Medicine,* Bantam Books.

———————— (1994). *Ageless Body, Timeless Mind: The Quantum Alternative to Growing Old,* Three Rivers Press.

Cole, Christopher R., et. al. (1999). "Heart-Rate Recovery Immediately after Exercise as a Predictor of Mortality," *New England Journal of Medicine,* Volume 341:1351–1357, October 28.

Conrad, Claudius, et. al. (2007). "Overture for Growth Hormone: Requiem for Interleukin-6," *Critical Care in Medicine,* Vol. 35, No. 12.

Cousins, Norman (1979). *Anatomy of an Illness as Perceived by the Patient: Reflections on Healing and Regeneration,* Norton. Introduction by Rene Dubos.

Davidson, R. J. (1995). "Cerebral asymmetry, emotion and affective style," in *Brain Asymmetry* (Richard. J. Davidson and Kenneth Hugdahl, eds.), MIT Press.

Doidge, Norman (2007). *The Brain That Changes Itself: Stories of Personal Triumph from the Frontiers of Brain Science,* Penguin Books.

Duncan, John Charles (1946). *Astronomy: A Textbook,* Harper & Brothers.

Edinger, Edward F. (1985). *Anatomy of the Psyche,* Open Court Publishing Company.

Egolf, B. (1992). "The Roseto effect: A 50-year comparison of mortality rates," *American Journal of Public Health,* August; 82(8), 1089–1092.

Erikson, Erik H. (1977). *Childhood and Society. Revised.* London: Triad/Paladin.

Evans-Wentz, W. Y., ed. (1971). Jung, *The Tibetan Book of the Great Liberation,* Oxford University Press.

Fordham, Michael (1985). *Explorations into the Self,* published for the Society of Analytical Psychology, Karnac Books.

Forryan, Barbara and Janet M. Glover (1979). *General Index to the Collected Works of C. G. Jung.* Bollingen Series, Vol. 20, Princeton University Press.

Foster, C. (2011). *Wired for God: The Biology of Spiritual Experience,* Hodder & Stoughton.

Franknoi, Andrew (2007). "How Fast are you Moving When you are Sitting Still?" *The Universe in the Classroom,* Spring.

Franz, Marie-Louise von (1974). *Number and Time: Reflections Leading towards a Unification of Psychology and Physics,* Rider & Co.

———— (2001). *Creation Myths,* Shambhala.

———— (1997). *Alchemical Active Imagination,* revised sub-edition, Shambhala.

Friedman, Richard A. (2002). "Like Drugs, Talk Therapy Can Change Brain Chemistry," *New York Times,* August 27.

Gartner, John D. (2005). *The Hypomaniac Edge,* Simon & Schuster.

Gill, Lisa (2008). "Music Provides Healing Grace Note for Hospital Patients," *USA Today,* June 17.

Goldapple, Kimberly, et. al. (2004). "Modulation of Cortical-Limbic Pathways in Major Depression: Treatment-Specific Effects of Cognitive Behavior Therapy," *Archives of General Psychiatry,* 61.

Grechko, Olga (2009). "Visual Stimuli Generated by Biochemical Reactions: Discrete Chaotic Dynamics as a Basis for Neurofeedback," *Journal of Neurotherapy.*

Gurnaratana, Shree Bhante Henepola (2001). *Eight Mindful Steps to Happiness; Walking the Buddha's Path,* Wisdom Publications.

Haekel, Ernst (1900). *The Riddle of the Universe,* translated by J. McCabe, Harper.

Haeffner, Mark (1991). *The Dictionary of Alchemy: From Maria Prophetissa to Isaac Newton,* Aquarian Press.

Hall, Calvin S. and Vernon J. Nordby (1972). *The Individual and His Dreams,* New American Library.

Hamer, D. H. (2005). *The God Gene: How Faith Is Hardwired into Our Genes,* Anchor Press.

Hannah, Barbara (1999). *The Inner Journey: Lectures and Essays on Jungian Psychology,* Inner City Books.

Hebb, D. O. (1949). *The Organization of Behavior,* Wiley.

Henderson, P. G., D. H. Rosen, and N. Mascaro (2007). "Empirical study on the healing nature of mandalas," *Psychology of Aesthetics, Creativity, and the Arts*, 1, 148–154.

Howell, Alice O. (1987). *Jungian Symbolism in Astrology*, American Federation of Astrologers, 4th edition.

Horne-Thomson, Anne and Denise Grocke (2008). "The Effect of Music Therapy on Anxiety in Patients who are Terminally Ill," *Journal of Palliative Medicine*, May.

Iyengar, B. K. S. (1985). *Light on Pranayama: The Yogic Art of Breathing*, Crossroad Publishing Company.

————— (2001). *Light on Yoga*, Thorsons Publishers.

Jacobi, Jalonde (1951). *The Psychology of C. G. Jung*, Yale University Press.

James, William (1988). *The Varieties of Religious Experience*, in *Writings: A Study in Human Nature Being the Gifford Lectures on Natural Religion Delivered at Edinburgh in 1901–1902*, (Classic Reprint), Library of America Publishers.

Jayakar, Pupul (1985). *Aditi: The Living Arts of India*, Smithsonian Institution Press.

Johnson, Robert A. (1989). *Inner Work: Using Dreams and Active Imagination for Personal Growth*, HarperOne.

Joshua, C. A. (2005). "Humor and oncology," *Journal of Clinical Oncology*, 23, 645–648.

Jung, C. G. (2009). *The Red Book: Liber Novus*, Philemon Series, W. W. Norton and Company. Edited and introduced by Sonu Shamdasani.

————— (1996). *The Psychology of Kundalini Yoga*. Bollingen Series, Princeton University Press. Notes of the seminar given in 1932 by C. G. Jung, edited by Sonu Shamdasani.

————— (1989). *Confrontation with the Unconscious in Memories, Dreams and Reflections*, Vintage Books. Edited by Aniela Jaffe.

————— (1984). *Seminar on Dream Analysis*, Bollingen Series, Princeton University Press. Compiled by William McGuire.

————— (1981a). *The Development of Personality*, in *The Collected Works of C. G. Jung*, Vol. 17, Routledge & Kegan Paul.

——————— (1981b). *Freud and Psychoanalysis,* in *The Collected Works of C. G. Jung,* Vol. 4, Routledge & Kegan Paul.

——————— (1981c). *Psychological Types,* in *The Collected Works of C. G. Jung,* Vol. 6, Routledge & Kegan Paul.

——————— (1976). *The Symbolic Life: Miscellaneous Writings,* Bollingen Series, Vol. 18, Princeton University Press.

——————— (1973). *Experimental Researches,* in *The Collected Works of C. G. Jung,* Vol. 2, Princeton University Press.

——————— (1970a). *Civilization in Transition,* in *The Collected Works of C. G. Jung,* 2nd ed., Vol. 10, Princeton University Press.

——————— (1970b). *Mysterium Coniunctionis: An Inquiry into the Separation and Synthesis of Psychic Opposites* in *Alchemy,* Bollingen Series, Vol. 14, Princeton University Press.

——————— (1969a). *The Archetypes and the Collective Unconscious, Part 1,* in *The Collected Works of C. G. Jung,* 2nd ed., Vol. 1, Princeton University Press.

——————— (1969b). *The Structure and Dynamics of the Psyche,* in *The Collected Works of C. G. Jung,* Vol. 8, Princeton University Press.

——————— (1968a). *Alchemical Studies,* in *The Collected Works of C. G. Jung,* Vol. 13, Routledge & Kegan Paul.

——————— (1968b). *Psychology and Alchemy,* in *The Collected Works of C. G. Jung,* 2nd ed., Vol. 12, Routledge & Kegan Paul; Princeton University Press.

——————— (1966a). *The Practice of Psychotherapy: Essays on the Psychology of the Transference and Other Subjects,* in *The Collected Works of C. G. Jung,* Vol. 16, Princeton University Press.

——————— (1966b). *The Spirit in Man, Art, and Literature,* Bollingen Series, Vol 15, Pantheon Books.

——————— (1960). *The Psychogenesis of Mental Disease,* in *The Collected Works of C. G. Jung,* Vol 3, Routledge & Kegan Paul.

——————— (1959). *Aion, Researches into the Phenomenology of the Self,* Part 2, Bollingen Series, Vol. 9, Pantheon Books.

——————— (1958). *Psychology and Religion: West and East,* in *The Collected Works of C. G. Jung,* Vol. 11, Routledge & Kegan Paul.

——————— (1957). *Psychiatric Studies,* Volume 1, Bollingen Series, Vol. 1, Pantheon Books.

————— (1957). *The Tibetan Book of the Dead* (W. Y. Evans-Wentz, ed.) Psychological Commentary by C. G. Jung, Oxford University Press.

————— (1956). *Symbols of Transformation: An Analysis of the Prelude to a Case of Schizophrenia,* Bollingen Series, 2nd ed., Vol. 5, Princeton University Press.

Jung, C. G. and R. F. C. Hull (1966). *Two Essays on Analytical Psychology,* Bollingen Series, Vol. 7. Princeton University Press.

Jung, C. G. and Lisa Ress (1979). *General Bibliography of C. G. Jung's Writings,* Bollingen Series, Vol. 19, Princeton University Press.

Kabat-Zinn, Jon (1990). *Full Catastrophe Living: Using the Wisdom of Your Body and Mind to Face Stress, Pain and Illness,* Bantam Dell.

Kalsched, Donald (1996). *The Inner World of Trauma: Archetypal Defenses of the Personal Spirit,* Routledge.

Kandel, E. R. (2009). "The Biology of Memory: A Forty-Year Perspective," *Journal of Neuroscience* 29: 12748–12756.

Kark, G. S. (1996). "Does religious observance promote health? Mortality in secular vs religious kibbutzim in Israel," *American Journal of Public Health,* 86:3, 341–346.

Keating, Thomas (2009). *Intimacy with God: An Introduction to Centering Prayer,* 3rd edition, Crossroad Publishing Company.

Kinsley, David (1986). *Hindu Goddesses, Visions of the Divine Feminine in the Hindu Religious Tradition,* University of California Press.

Kraft, Ulrich (2006). "Train Your Brain," *Scientific American Mind,* February 1.

Leadbetter, Ron (1997). *Encyclopedia Mythica,* "Hermes," *www.pantheon.org/articles.*

Lutz, A., et. al. (2004). "Long-term meditators self-induce high-amplitude gamma synchrony during mental practice," *Proceedings of the National Academy of Sciences,* 101.

MacLean, Paul D. (1990). *The Triune Brain in Evolution: Role in Paleocerebral Functions,* Springer Publications.

Martin, Stephen D. et al. (2001). "Brain Blood Flow Changes in Depressed Patients Treated with Interpersonal Psychotherapy or

Venlafaxine Hydrochloride: Preliminary Findings," *Archives of General Psychiatry*, July 01, 58(7):641–648.

Matthews, Boris, ed. (1986). *The Herder Symbol Dictionary*, Chiron Publications.

Nippoldt, Todd (2011). "Is There Such a Thing as Adrenal Fatigue?" *mayoclinic.com*.

Ouspensky, P. D. (1922). *Tertium Organum: The Third Canon of Thought, A Key to the Enigmas of the World*, 2nd edition, translated by Nicholas Bessaraboff and Claude Bragdon, Alfred A. Knopf.

Pennington, Basil (1982). "Centering Prayer: Renewing an Ancient Christian Prayer Form," *Image*, August 17.

Penson, P. R. (2005). "Laughter: the best medicine?" *Oncologist*, 10, 651–660.

Perry, John Weir (1974). *The Far Side of Madness*, Spring Publications.

Pintchman, Tracy (1994). *The Rise of the Goddess in Hindu Tradition*, State University of New York Press.

Preyer, William (1888/1909). *The Mind of the Child*, Vol. 1 and 2, translated by W. Brown, Appleton.

Ramos, Denise Gimenez (2004). *The Psyche of the Body—A Jungian Approach to Psychosomatics,* Brunner-Routledge.

Randolph, C. and M. Byrd (1988). "Positive Therapeutic Effects of Intercessory Prayer in a Coronary Care Unit Population," *Southern Medical Journal*, 81:7, 826–829.

Ratnayake, Shantha. "Meditation Sharpens the Mind, Attention, and the Distribution of Neural Resources," *www.mindupdate.com*.

Reh, F. "John Pareto's Principle: The 80/20 Rule: How the 80/20 Rule can help you be More Effective," *www.About.com*.

Rosen, David H. (1993). *Transforming Depression: A Jungian Approach Using Creative Art,* Jeremy P. Tarcher-Putnam Book.

Rosen, David H., N. Mascaro, R. Arnau, M. Escamilla, M. Tai-Seale, C. Sanders, P. Henderson, U. Hoang, and K. Stephenson (2010). "Depression in Medical Students: Gene-Environment Interactions," *Annals of Behavioral Science and Medical Education*, 16, 2:8–14.

Rosen, M. with S. Brenner (2003). *Rosen method bodywork: Accessing the unconscious through touch*, North Atlantic Books.

Sackeim, H. A., et. al. (2006). "Durability of Antidepressant Response to Vagus Nerve Stimulation," *International Journal of Neuropsychopharmacology*, October.

Sarkamo, Teppo, et. al. (2008). "Music Listening Enhances Cognitive Recovery and Mood after Middle Cerebral Artery Stroke," *Brain* 131, 866–867.

Seaward, B. L. (1992). "Humor's healing potential," *Health Programs*, 1992; 73, 66–70.

Spiegel, David M. (2003). "Utilization of Integrative Medicine," National Center for Complementary Medicine presentation, *nccam.nih.gov/training/videolectures/mindbody*.

Spiegelman, J. Marvin and Arwind U. Vasavada (1987). *Hinduism and Jungian Psychology*, Falcon Press.

Srinivasan, K. (2006). "Heart Rate Variability and Psychiatry: Beyond Heart-Mind Link," presented at the 156th American Psychiatric Association annual meeting, May 20–25, Toronto, Canada.

Stevens, Anthony (2005). *The Two-Million-Year-Old Self*, in *Carolyn and Ernest Fay Series in Analytical Psychology,* foreword by David Rosen, Texas A & M University Press.

Wampold, Bruce E., et al. (1997). "A Meta-Analysis of Outcome Studies Comparing Bona Fide Psychotherapies: Empirically, All Must Have Prizes," *Psychological Bulletin*, Vol. 122.

W., Bill (1988). "The Language of the Heart," in *Bill W.'s Grapevine Writings*, AA Grapevine Inc.

Waldman, A. N. and Newberg A. (2009). *How God Changes Your Brain: Breakthrough Findings from a Leading Neuroscientist*, Ballantine Books.

Weisenberg, M. T. I. (1995). "Humor as a cognitive technique for increasing pain tolerance," *Pain*, 63, 207–212.

Wulsin, Lawson (2009). "Autonomic Imbalance, Depression and Coronary Artery Disease: Facing our Scotoma," presented at the American Psychiatric Association's annual meeting, May 21, San Francisco.

Ziegler, Jan (1995). "Immune System May Benefit from the Ability to Laugh," *Journal of the National Cancer Institute*, Oxford University Press, March 1, 1995; 87(5): 342–343.

Primary Sources and Ancient Texts:

Athara-Veda-Samhita, translated by W. D. Whitney and Bhasya of Sayancharya, edited and revised by K. L. Joshi, Indica Books, Varanasi 2000 (originally *The Harvard Oriental Series*, Vol. 7–8, 1905).

Bhagavad Gita, translated by Edwin Arnold, Dover Publications, 1993.

Hymns of Atharva Veda, 2 Volumes, translated by Ralph T. H. Griffith. Chowkhamba Sanskrit Series, no. 66. Varanasi: Chowkhamba Sanskrit Series Office, 1968.

Rig Veda-Samhita; together with the commentary of Sayanacharya, edited by F. Max Muller, 1st Indian edition, 4 volumes. Chowkhamba Sanskrit Series, no. 99. Varanasi: Chowkhamba Sanskrit Series Office, 1966.

Translations of the Vedic Hymns, Sacred Books of the East, Vol. 32, translated by F. Max Muller. Delhi: Motilal Banarsidas, Reprint 1964.

Vajasaneyi-Samhita in Maadhyandina and Knave Sakha, with the commentary of Mahidhara, 2nd edition, edited by Albrecht Weber. Chowkhamba Sanskrit Series, no. 1003.

White Yajur Veda, translated by Ralph R. H. Griffith. Varanasi: R. J. J. Lazarus and Company, 1899.

Yajur Veda, translated by Devi Chand. New Delhi: S. Paul and Co., 1965.

Yajurveda Samhita, translated by Ralph T. H. Griffith. Delhi Nag Publishers, 1990.

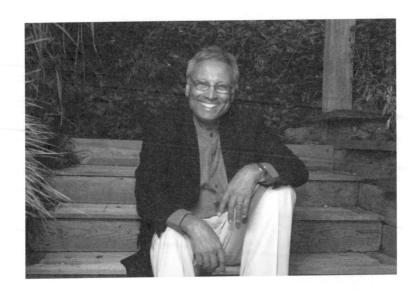

About the Author

Ashok Bedi is a Jungian psychoanalyst and a board-certified psychiatrist. He is a member of the Royal College of Psychiatrists of Great Britain, a Diplomat in Psychological Medicine at the Royal College of Physicians and Surgeons of England, and a Distinguished Life Fellow of the American Psychiatric Association. He is a Clinical Professor in Psychiatry at the Medical College of Wisconsin in Milwaukee and president, training analyst, and faculty member at the Analyst Training Program of the Carl G. Jung Institute of Chicago. He practices psychiatry at the Aurora Psychiatric Hospital and the Aurora Health Care Network, and has been a psychiatric consultant to several agencies in Metro Milwaukee. Presently, Dr. Bedi is a consultant for the Sexual Assault Treatment Center at the Aurora Sinai Samaritan Hospital and at the Dewey Center of the Aurora Psychiatric Hospital for Treatment of Addictions, as well as for the Pastoral Counseling Service of Greater Milwaukee.

Trained in India, Great Britain, and the United States, Dr. Bedi is interested in the emerging frontiers of spirituality and healing, and the synapses of the mind, body, soul, and Spirit. He is author of *Path to the Soul* (Weiser Books, 2000) and *Awaken the Slumbering Goddess: The Latent Code of the Hindu Goddess Archetypes* (Booksurge Publishers, 2007), and coauthor of *Retire Your Family Karma* (Nicholas-Hays, Inc., 2003). These and his other upcoming presentations can be previewed at his website, *www.pathtothesoul.com*.

Dr. Bedi has been in practice in Milwaukee for over thirty years, specializing in adult psychotherapy and Jungian psychoanalysis. He regularly presents lectures and seminars in India, Great Britain, Ireland, and the United States on the spiritual and analytical dimensions of treatment, healing, and personal growth. Over the last several years, he has been liaison for the International Association of Analytical Psychologists charged with developing Jungian training programs in India. He travels annually to India to teach, train, and consult with Jungian groups at several centers, including in Mumbai, Ahmedabad, and Bangalore. He leads the annual "In the Footsteps of Carl Jung in India" study group to several centers there under the auspices of the New York Jung Foundation.